Up to LOSE 10 POUNDS in 2 WEEKS
POCKET GUIDE

Dedicated to the millions of people
who are committed to losing weight.
May you live a happy and healthy life.

By Alex A. Llu... ...rt
Author of C...

WS Publishing Group
www.WSPublishingGroup.com
San Diego, California

Lose Up to 10 Pounds in 2 Weeks Pocket Guide
By Alex A. Lluch

Copyright © 2012 by WS Publishing Group, Inc.
San Diego, California

Nutritional and fitness guidelines based on information provided by the United States Food and Drug Administration, Food and Nutrition Information Center, National Agricultural Library, Agricultural Research Service, and the U.S. Department of Agriculture.

For more best-selling titles by WS Publishing Group,
visit www.wspublishinggroup.com

Exercise photos:
Tawn Tu, www.knightphotovideo.com
Aaron Tsai, www.aaroneye.com
Models:
Brettan Bablove & David Defenbaugh

ISBN: 978-1-936061-40-2

Printed in China

contents

contents

Introduction

You know the frightening statistics by now: Sixty-seven percent of Americans are overweight, with 34 percent being considered obese. Millions of people are struggling with their weight every day and suffering the effects, from lack of energy to infertility to diabetes to heart disease. Perhaps most tangible, however, are the feelings of frustration, disappointment and self-doubt that trying to lose weight and failing bring. And many times, the last 10 pounds are the most difficult and stressful to lose. You may have already lost a great deal of weight but are struggling with a particularly stubborn 10 pounds. Or, you may be very close to your ideal weight, but having a hard time jumpstarting your metabolism or getting the motivation to lose the extra 10 pounds.

That's because so many diets are doomed to fail. They either force you to go cold turkey with the foods you love (causing cravings and bingeing), tell you to substitute real food with an unappealing powdered drink or meal replacement bar, or promote fast and easy weight loss through eating only certain foods and eliminating whole food groups (read: the lemonade-and-cayenne pepper diet or the grapefruit diet; extremely unhealthy). None of these types of diets are healthy or sustainable, meaning you'll only gain the weight right back afterward. And you're not learning any new eating or exercise habits, so you'll simply revert back to your old lifestyle, the one that made you gain weight in the first place.

The *Lose Up to 10 Pounds in 2 Weeks Pocket Guide* diet and fitness program, however, is full of the most powerful, proven secrets in the world to help you lose the weight you want in record time. Slim down for a class reunion, vacation, birthday celebration, or just because swimsuit season is never far off. Or maybe there's no special occasion; maybe you're just tired of carrying around 10 or more extra pounds and you know, with a little dedication and several fast lifestyle changes, you can be at weight you want. Being healthier, happier and in better shape with more energy are always the best reasons for losing weight. Medical research has shown that losing just 5 to 10 percent of your body weight can significantly improve a person's health by lowering cholesterol and the risk of heart disease, stroke and diabetes.

What's interesting about this program is that the amount of weight you're trying to lose is a deceptive amount — it's not 100 pounds, it's about 10. Seems like it should be easy, right? Well, of course it's not. Someone who needs to lose 100 pounds burns many more calories just by going through his or her day with all that extra weight. But someone who is slimmer, who wants to lose just a few pounds, is burning far fewer calories than a heavier person. Consider running on a treadmill for an hour — when you start, the machine requires you to enter your weight. That is because an hour of running at the same intensity burns many fewer calories for someone who is 150 pounds, than for someone who is 200 pounds. Additionally, as we age and our metabolisms slow down, the body gets comfortable with the extra pounds and it's tougher to lose them. Your body needs a jumpstart, just like a car with a stalled battery! You'll find the diet and fitness tips in this book to be just what you need to get moving more efficiently, cooking smarter, planning ahead, and eating better. And unlike other diets, where you're eliminating the nutrients your body truly needs, you won't be starving or exhausted. This program is what is considered a "flexible diet," one that instructs dieters to monitor the consumption of calories to lose weight. You won't starve, eat only one kind of food or miss out on dinners with friends or your favorite treats — you just need to implement the diet and fitness secrets you'll learn in this book and keep your eye on the prize — losing up to 10 pounds!

The heart of the *Lose Up to 10 Pounds in 2 Weeks Pocket Guide* program includes three basic steps:

1   Using a formula to determine the calories your body burns at rest, or your BMR

2   Tracking everything you eat and all the physical activity you do daily for 2 weeks

3   Creating a substantial daily caloric deficit — meaning that you are expending more calories than you take in through a combination of eating less and burning calories with exercise. The larger the calorie deficit you create each day, the more weight you will lose.

At the end of each day, you will add up the calories you ate and drank. Then you'll take the resulting number and subtract the calories burned from physical activity to calculate your Net Calories. Next, subtract your BMR (the calories your body burns at rest) to find your daily total calorie deficit. You can find a detailed example of this formula in the section called "Journal Pages."

In addition, with this program you will mentally create a calorie "budget" for each meal and snack, which means anticipating how many calories you need to save and preparing for each meal with a set amount to spend in mind. For example, you might budget 400 calories for lunch. You can have any meal and drink you want, as long as you stay within your budget. And, if it's possible to save a few calories by eating less than the budgeted amount, you can save up for the next meal or do slightly less exercise to lose even more weight!

If it sounds like a big change and hard work, that's because it is. No one is going to pretend it will be easy. You will have to make major changes, like cutting out empty carbs and calories, eating more fruits and vegetables and whole grains, and building fitness into your life every day. But the results will be worth it. Fitting into that favorite dress again, seeing the look on an old boyfriend's face, lounging on the beach in a swimsuit without feeling anxious — you will be highly rewarded for your hard work over the next 2 weeks and beyond.

By purchasing this book, you have taken the first step in your weight-loss journey to looking and feeling amazing. In just 2 weeks, you could be 10 pounds lighter!

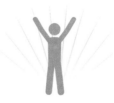

How to Use This Book

Congratulations! You've taken the first step toward losing real weight in a short amount of time by getting all the tools you need. Portable and a convenient size, this book easily slips in a purse, briefcase or gym bag so you will always have these weight-loss secrets at your fingertips.

This book offers you many valuable tools and features for cutting calories, getting in great shape, and successfully meeting your weight-loss goals, including:

Filling out your personal health and fitness profile

Before you begin the *Lose Up to 10 Pounds in 2 Weeks* program, you need to build Your Personal Profile. This section helps you assess your current physical state, habits, and preferences for diet and exercise. With this information, you will be able to determine where you started and how far you've come, as well as identify your goals and any potential obstacles.

In this section you will also determine the optimum amount of calories, fat and carbs that you will aim to eat every day.

Determining your BMR and creating a daily calorie deficit

An important part of the *Lose Up to 10 Pounds in 2 Weeks Pocket Guide* program is calculating your basal metabolic rate, or BMR. Your BMR is the number of calories your body would burn naturally, even if you didn't move all day. Knowing this number is the first step to this program because it's how you build a calorie deficit.

Each day, you will total up the amount of calories you have eaten and subtract the calories you have burned from physical activity to find your Net Calorie Total. In order to lose up to 10 pounds in this short time, you need to create a substantial calorie deficit each day, through a combination of diet and exercise. For example, one day, you may be able to cut 500 calories out of your diet, and then also burn 500 calories through exercise to create a 1,000-calorie deficit. Once you create a 3,500-calorie deficit, you will have lost 1 pound.

Powerful diet secrets and tips, fast places to trim calories, motivational quotes, and more

Each chapter and section of this book is packed with the secrets of cutting calories, making lifestyle changes, and losing weight. You will learn to boost your metabolism, make healthier eating decisions, as well as one of the best weight-loss strategies around: developing a game plan for avoiding pitfalls and sticking to your daily calorie goals. Throughout this book you will practice conscious eating, curb your appetite, and stop sabotaging your weight-loss efforts. You will also learn to anticipate and recognize situations that cause you to binge or eat unhealthy foods and pinpoint the emotions and triggers that cause you to overeat.

You will recognize the changes you can make without starving or depriving yourself, because no diet and fitness plan is going to work if you're feeling lethargic and hungry all the time. Burning hundreds of calories more than you take in a day might sound difficult, that's why each chapter in this book is complete with Did You Know facts and quick and easy places to trim 100, 200, and 300 or more calories. You'll discover new ways to eat less and lose weight that you never even thought of!

Ultimate fitness secrets for burning calories and body fat and staying motivated

Fitness is going to be the second key to losing up to 10 pounds. You can't do it with diet alone! These chapters will give you all the tips, tricks and tools to maximize each and every workout and physical activity you do. You'll get insight into everything from fitness basics to little-known secrets of getting in shape quickly and without burning out.

In the Activities & Calories Burned chapter, you'll see that calories are burned in all sorts of ways, from sports to casual physical activity to normal household chores. This section that will be a great asset in finding the sports and activities that you can make a part of your daily routine to burn calories.

Powerful 14-day exercise program for maximum weight loss

The fitness section also includes a detailed exercise program that combines a strength training circuit with a cardio circuit six days out of the week to burn calories and body fat quickly. The plan is designed to be done anywhere, so you won't need any props or weights. You will switch off each day between an upper body and core strength training circuit and a lower body and core strength training circuit. Each day, you will also alternate between a plyometric cardio circuit and a kickboxing cardio circuit. The last day of the week is to rest, recuperate and relax.

Use your number one weight-loss tool!

People who keep a food and fitness journal are proven to lose *twice* as much weight as those who don't. As you read all the valuable, powerful weight-loss and fitness tips in this book, you will be keeping track of what you eat and drink in the journal in the back of the book. Each daily page lets you write down the food and beverages you have daily, as well as the physical activities you do to burn calories. You'll easily be able to see what you've eaten and, thus, plan ahead for each meal and workout.

Keeping a diet journal will most likely be a healthy reality check. Studies have shown that people tend to dramatically underestimate the number of calories in the foods they eat — by as much as 50 percent! The diet and fitness journal portion of this book allows you to break down your caloric intake by meal and item to get real about exactly how many calories you're consuming. Once you recognize the high-calorie foods in your diet, you can replace some things with lower calorie options or cut back on portion sizes. Additionally, having your food intake right in front of you keeps you accountable — because who wants to look back and see the hundreds of calories from a pizza-and-cheese-bread binge written in their journal? You'll think twice before indulging in a huge or highly caloric meal. The journal will also help keep you motivated to exercise daily and provide a place to record your weight as the numbers on the scale begin to drop.

Your Personal Profile

Begin your program by gathering some information to assess your current physical state, habits, and preferences.

Fill in the information on the following pages. Visit your primary care physician and have your cholesterol, triglycerides, and blood pressure measured. These levels will also factor into the choices you make when creating your diet and fitness plan. You should also take your current measurements and place a "Before" photo in this section. It will be motivating to look back and see a visual of where you began and how far you have come.

Next, assess your diet and fitness history. You will also answer some questions about your past attempts to lose weight and what obstacles you encountered. Finally, outline your goals. Determine what you hope to accomplish with this program, which types of physical activities you most enjoy, and your intake goals, including the specific amounts of calories, fats, and carbs your diet should include daily.

Good luck meeting all your goals!

Your Health Profile

Complete the following personal health profile. You can request necessary information from your primary health care provider.

Name: _____   Triglycerides: _____

Age: _____   HDL Cholesterol: _____

Height: _____   LDL Cholesterol: _____

Total cholesterol: _____   Blood Pressure: _____

Current Physical Activity: (sedentary, moderately active, very active)

_____

_____

_____

Current Diet & Eating Habits: (fast food, snack often, late-night eating, etc.)

_____

_____

_____

Other Current Habits: (smoking, drinking, lack of sleep, etc.)

_____

_____

_____

DATE: _____ WEIGHT: _____ BODY FAT %: _____

MEASUREMENTS:

|_____| chest |_____| biceps |_____| waist |_____| hips |_____| thighs

tape your photo here

PHOTO COMMENTS: _____

Dietary Habits Questionnaire

The following questions will assist you in developing your weight-loss program.

Which best describes your daily eating habits?
- ❏ Three average meals
- ❏ Graze frequently
- ❏ One large meal, little else

What types of food do you crave the most?
- ❏ Meat/fish
- ❏ Fruit/vegetables
- ❏ Bread/cereals/rice
- ❏ Sweets

Do you typically eat out or prepare food for yourself?
- ❏ I usually cook my food
- ❏ I eat out or have premade meals

What is your weight-loss goal?
- ❏ Lose 10 or more pounds
- ❏ Maintain weight
- ❏ Lose a little weight
- ❏ Improve health

Which habits do you have?
- ❏ Skipping meals
- ❏ Drinking full-sugar soda
- ❏ Carb addiction
- ❏ Overeating while dining out

Describe your body type:
- ❏ Overweight
- ❏ Average
- ❏ Muscular

For what particular event (if any) do you want to lose weight?

_____

_____

_____

What is your number one reason for wanting to lose weight?

_____

_____

_____

_____

Your Diet & Intake Goals

A huge part of your weight-loss journey will be managing your diet and intake. Record your goals here and use them as a barometer for what you eat every day.

YOUR DIET GOALS

_____

_____

_____

_____

_____

_____

YOUR INTAKE GOALS

Based on the number of calories your diet allows, list the daily targets that you would like to meet. (Your primary care physician can also help you determine the appropriate amounts.)

DAILY CALORIES: **FAT gms:**   **CARBS gms:**   **OTHER:** _____

NOTES: _____

_____

_____

Your Fitness History

It is important to look back at your past experiences with getting in shape and losing weight to determine the diet and workout plan that will have the greatest chance for success.

Is there any reason why you should not engage in physical activity?

At what age were you in your best physical shape?

Have you ever participated in a workout program? When?

How long did you stay with the program?

What did the program include?

What led you to or inspired you to get into shape now?

What obstacles have kept you from meeting your fitness goals?

What will ensure these obstacles do not inhibit you this time?

Rate your current fitness level on a scale of 1-10
(1=Worst 10=Best).

Workout Plan Questionnaire

A successful fitness plan is one that includes activities you enjoy. Be honest in answering the following questions and you will be able to develop a plan you can maintain.

Which types of physical activity do you enjoy participating in?

❏ Aerobics
❏ Active gardening
❏ Backpacking
❏ Baseball/softball
❏ Bicycling/spinning
❏ Climbing
❏ Cross country skiing
❏ Dancing
❏ Downhill skiing
❏ Football
❏ Golfing
❏ Hiking
❏ Hockey
❏ Jogging/running
❏ Jump roping

❏ Martial arts
❏ Pilates
❏ Racquetball/handball
❏ Roller blading
❏ Rowing
❏ Soccer
❏ Skating
❏ Stair/bench stepping
❏ Stretching
❏ Swimming
❏ Tennis
❏ Volleyball
❏ Walking
❏ Weight training
❏ Yoga

How many times a week do you want to work out?

❏ 1-2 days   ❏ 2-3 days   ❏ 3-4 days   ❏ 5+ days

How long will each session be, on average?

❏ 10-20 minutes
❏ 20-30 minutes
❏ 30-45 minutes

❏ 45-60 minutes
❏ 60-90 minutes
❏ 90+ minutes

Your Fitness Goals

By first identifying your goals, you can create a specific workout routine to help you achieve them. Your goals should be specific, quantifiable, realistic and time-based. Fill out the following questions honestly and with a critical eye. You'll be able to use the resulting information to get inspired and ward off possible pitfalls.

What do you want to accomplish with your workout program?
(Check the boxes next to the goals that are most important to you.)

❑ Improve cardiovascular fitness and endurance

❑ Improve diet and or eating habits

❑ Improve flexibility

❑ Improve health

❑ Improve strength

❑ Improve muscle tone and shape

❑ Increase energy

❑ Lose weight

❑ Prevent injury and/or

❑ Rehabilitate injury

❑ Train for a sports-specific event

❑ Reduce cholesterol

❑ Reduce blood pressure

❑ Reduce risk of disease

❑ Reduce stress

❑ Gain weight

❑ Other: _____

❑ Other: _____

What types of physical activity do you like and dislike?

_____

_____

Do you prefer to exercise alone, with a partner, or in a group?

_____

_____

Calculating Your BMR

Knowing your basal metabolic rate, or BMR, is crucial to this program. Your BMR is the number of calories your body burns naturally, at rest. Your BMR is based on your age, height and current weight and decreases with age, meaning that it becomes harder to lose weight and keep it off as you get older. However, with a healthy diet and fitness plan, you can increase your BMR and lose weight more easily.

Use these formulas to calculate your BMR, then use this number in your daily diet and fitness journal pages.

Female BMR = 655 + (4.3 x weight in pounds) + (4.7 x height in inches) - (4.7 x age in years)

Male BMR = 66 + (6.3 x weight in pounds) + (12.9 x height in inches) - (6.8 x age in years)

Your BMR:

> **❝** The great thing in the world is not so much where we stand, as in what direction we are moving. **❞**

~ Oliver Wendell Holmes

Chapter 1

Changing the Way You Live

Losing weight takes a tremendous effort. If it were an easy thing to do, everyone would be at their perfect weight. When you talk about a body and lifestyle makeover, you can feel yourself getting excited, but when it comes time to actually implement the changes, your to-do list feels so long that you get overwhelmed and give up. Or, in the past you might have made it a few weeks into a weight-loss plan, failed to see results and quit. It's natural for the body to resist change. Your body tries to protect itself by slowing its basal metabolism, the rate at which you burn calories while at rest, making weight loss difficult. However, this program will have you looking and feeling better immediately, starting with the simple lifestyle changes in the chapter. Read through them and commit yourself to implementing them. They are what your body and mind need to jumpstart your weight loss, give you more energy, and get you motivated to complete the 2-week program.

Mahatma Gandhi once said, "Be the change you want to see in the world." Being healthier and living better are goals everyone should strive for. You will likely find that after living the *Lose Up to 10 Pounds in 2 Weeks* program, you won't want to stop! You'll feel better and slimmer than ever before, and you won't want to go back to old habits that packed on the extra pounds. However, even if you don't continue beyond this 2-week program, know that all the changes you'll find in this book are sustainable for a lifetime. This book gives you the tools to lose 10 pounds in 2 weeks, and more, including powerful, proven diet and exercise secrets and tips, motivational quotes, a custom fitness plan, and, the ultimate weight-loss tool, a daily diet and fitness journal. With all this at your fingertips, it's just up to you to put everything into practice.

Losing up to 10 pounds in 2 weeks starts by modifying your everyday habits. Today, you get a clean slate to erase the past and create a new, healthier, thinner way of living.

Keep your eye on the prize

Staying motivated is all about determining the top reasons you want and need to lose weight and reminding yourself on the days you're tempted to eat a high-calorie dessert or skip the gym. Are you losing weight to look and feel great at a special event that is 2 weeks away, such as a high school reunion, wedding, vacation or birthday? Or did your doctor advise you that losing 10 pounds will help reduce your risk of disease, lower your blood pressure, or help you get pregnant? Are you looking forward to the increased amount of energy you'll have after losing a few pounds? Or are you simply tired of feeling powerless to food? Make a short list of the top 3 reasons you are losing 10 pounds. Hang this list where you can see it every day to remind you, along with a motivational image — a gorgeous beach, a dress you'd like to buy in a smaller size, the hike you plan to take when you have more energy.

Create great new habits

Changing the way you live starts with building new, healthy habits that support your weight loss. Let's say you have the bad habit of eating empty-calorie candy and chocolate — replace it with a healthy habit. Instead of snacking on a candy bar when you are in the mood for something sweet, try having a 60-calorie pudding cup or a bowl of fresh strawberries with low-fat Cool Whip. Get in the habit of keeping those items in your kitchen instead of sugary snacks and you'll have made one awesome, positive change to your lifestyle! Focus on including the good behavior into your routine every day for a week until it becomes second nature.

This book gives you the tools to lose up to 10 pounds, and more, including powerful, proven diet and exercise secrets and tips, motivational quotes, a custom fitness plan, and, the ultimate weight-loss tool, a daily diet and fitness journal.

Eat from all 6 of the main food groups

There are six main food groups: grains, fruits, vegetables, dairy, meat and beans, and oils and sweets. Odds are, you've been overdoing it in some and avoiding others all together. For instance, less than 3.5 percent of American men and women eat the FDA-recommended amount of fruits and vegetables. Unfortunately, when food groups are short-changed, you do not receive the balance of protein, carbohydrates, and plant-based nutrients that your body needs. To kickstart a sluggish metabolism, maintain your energy and inspire the body to burn fat cells, you must eat a balanced diet. The better you eat, the better your body works and the faster you'll lose weight. And you'll find that it only takes a few short days for your body to stop craving fatty and sugary processed foods. Some foods that pack mega-nutrients include low-fat yogurt, spinach, salmon, berries, avocados, whole grains, bell peppers, and olive oil.

Did You Know?
Depending on your height and body fat percentage, losing 10 pounds could mean dropping as much as 2 clothing sizes!

Ransack your kitchen and pantry

Step 1: Get a big trash bag. Step 2: Open your cabinets, pantry, fridge and yes, even the hidden spots where you stash treats. Step 3: Throw every high-calorie, high-fat, sugary, salty, processed piece of food into your trash bag. Step 4: Take one last look in the bag before you toss the bag into a dumpster. Say goodbye to unhealthy, bloating, weight-gain-causing snacks and treats! Step 5: Feel inspired by your clean (perhaps nearly empty) cupboards and shelves. You now have a clean slate to start filling your kitchen with healthy foods. Likewise, cravings are very visual, so if you open your cupboards and don't see fatty foods, you won't constantly think about them.

Break the addiction to high-calorie food!

Did you realize that constantly treating yourself to high-calorie foods can lead to an actual addiction to these foods? Eating a high-calorie meal triggers the release of dopamine and other feel-good chemicals in the brain. However, a ground-breaking report from the 2009 meeting for the Society for Neuroscience showed that rats that were fed a high-calorie diet of items like bacon, sausage and cheesecake actually had diminished response in the pleasure centers of their brains over time. As the animals' brain reward circuits became less responsive, they continued to overeat and become more and more obese. Their brains actually began to mimic those of rats addicted to drugs as they became addicted to high-calorie foods! Break this cycle by eliminating these high-fat, high-calorie foods from your grocery list. If they're not in the house or in your desk, you won't be tempted. Don't even look at the dessert list at a restaurant. Simply imagining yourself eating a delicious crème brulee can trigger an intense craving.

Get some shuteye

> One study showed that lack of sleep can lead to eating an extra 900 calories a day.

Research has proven that adults who get 7 to 9 hours of sleep a night eat less during the day and are much less likely to be overweight. For one, when you're sleep-deprived the body produces more of the hormone that causes feelings of hunger. Being exhausted also means less willpower to resist the temptation of fatty and sugary foods.

One study showed that lack of sleep can lead to eating an extra 900 calories a day. Wow! Consider that cutting those 900 calories a day for a year would mean a weight loss of more than 90 pounds! To lose up to 10 pounds, you need to give your body the rest it needs. Try going to bed earlier and establishing a routine at night that is calming and gets you ready for deep sleep. For instance, things like being online or watching TV can disrupt your ability to fall asleep and stay asleep, so try reading for 30 minutes or taking a relaxing bath.

Back away from the TV

The National Weight Control Registry (NWCR) is an organization that studies the behavioral and psychological factors that contribute to weight loss and the maintenance of long-term weight loss. The NWCR tracks more than 5,000 individuals over the age of 18 who have maintained at least a 30-pound weight loss for one year or longer (although the average registry member has lost an average of 66 pounds and kept it off for 5.5 years), and

> ## Trim Up to 200 Calories!
> **Pass:** Croutons, or
> **Swap:** Pita instead of French bread on a sandwich

found that there are a few common threads among members. About 80 percent of members report eating breakfast daily and, naturally, almost all members report continuing to maintain a low-calorie, low-fat diet and doing high levels of activity but, additionally, 62 percent say they watch less than 10 hours of TV per week. By contrast, the average American watches 38 hours a week, almost 4 times that much. That's nearly as many hours as a full-time job!

Obviously, if you're spending numerous hours a day in front of the TV, you're not exercising. In addition, vegging out leads to overeating of unhealthy foods, out of boredom or for comfort. Who ever curled up on the couch with a salad? As National Weight Control Registry members prove, getting off the couch and away from the TV aids in real weight loss. You'll eat less, and the hours you were spending watching a *Seinfeld* marathon can now be spent hitting the gym, going for a walk with a friend, or otherwise being active outdoors.

Drink little to no alcohol

Alcohol makes losing 10 pounds in 2 weeks much tougher. For one, when you drink alcohol, that is what your body processes first, before fat, protein or carbs. Thus, alcohol slows down the fat-burning process. Also, a serving of alcohol contains at least 120 calories, and that number can skyrocket if you use sugary mixers. If you take in 120 calories from alcohol, you'll have to find another place to cut it, either with extra exercise or eating less at another meal. That can be very difficult since you're already going to be on a calorie-restricted diet.

Since the goal of this diet plan is to find fast and easy places to cut hundreds of calories, drinking alcohol is counterproductive. Plus, it's never smart or healthy to replace nutritious food with alcohol, which offers no nutrients. Also, liquids don't satisfy you or fill you up. In fact, alcohol does quite the opposite. Research has shown that alcohol not only decreases willpower, it may stimulate the appetite — specifically cravings for fatty and salty foods. Studies have shown as much as a 20 percent increase in calories consumed at a meal when alcohol was served beforehand. So, while it's tough to say no alcohol at all for 2 weeks, the argument against it is very strong. Most dieticians believe there is no place for alcohol in a reduced-calorie diet.

Studies have shown as much as a 20 percent increase in calories consumed at a meal when alcohol was served beforehand.

If If you do not change direction, you may end up where you are heading. **"**

~ Lao Tzu

Chapter 2

Maximizing Your Metabolism

We often hear about metabolism and its importance in helping us lose weight. But what exactly is metabolism, and how can you make yours work harder for you?

Metabolism is a series of chemical reactions that convert the food we eat into energy. This energy powers everything we do, from thinking to moving, healing, growing, and even aging. When you eat, you take in energy in the form of sugars (carbohydrates), proteins, and fats. But the body's cells cannot use energy in this form. So the body must break down these substances so the energy can be distributed to and used by the body's cells. Molecules in the digestive system called enzymes break down each substance differently: proteins are broken down into amino acids, fats are broken down into fatty acids, and carbohydrates are broken down into simple sugars, such as glucose. The process of breaking these substances down and using them for energy is metabolism.

Metabolism is a complicated chemical sequence, so it is easier to think of it in its most basic sense — metabolism is process that influences how easily you can gain and lose weight, or how easily you store or burn calories. The number of calories you are able to burn in a day depends on how high or low your metabolism is. Earlier in this book, you calculated your basal metabolic rate, or BMR. This is the rate at which your body burns calories while at rest. Everyone has a different BMR, which is largely inherited. You have probably heard friends lament, "Oh, I have the slowest metabolism in the world," or, "Have you seen how much so-and-so eats? She must have a super-fast metabolism." However, genetics don't determine everything when it comes to how quickly or slowly your body burns calories. You can actually change your BMR by doing certain activities and eating certain foods. For example, regular exercise can increase your body's BMR. Muscle burns 3 times as many calories as fat — about 6 calories per pound for muscle and only 2 calories per pound for fat. Therefore, every extra pound of muscle you put on burns 30 to 50 extra calories per day. Finally, your eating habits — the times at which you eat and your intake of protein or other metabolism-friendly foods — can also increase your BMR.

If you're trying to subsist on carrots, lettuce and chicken soup, you'll be too exhausted to do much of anything but sit on the couch.

Don't settle for a slow metabolism or use it as an excuse for why you can't lose weight. This chapter gives you all the tips and tricks for super-charging your metabolism, starting from the moment you wake up in the morning.

Eat breakfast

It's called "the most important meal of the day" for a reason, and eating breakfast is essential for weight loss. Your body is deprived of food during the night — you are literally taking a "break" to "fast." Consider that if you ate dinner the night before at 7 p.m., and you go all the way to lunch without eating, you'll have fasted for 17 hours or more! Your blood sugar will be extremely low, plus, when your body doesn't receive sufficient nutrients post-fast, it will function less efficiently. Eating a balanced breakfast jumpstarts your metabolism, helps you eat a normal portion at lunch, and provides blood-sugar stability that means more energy, brainpower and focus for your day. And no, a cup of coffee isn't breakfast. Whole grains, oats, peanut butter, fruit, low-fat yogurt, and eggs are all good ways to start your day. They get your metabolism kicking and prevent overeating throughout the day.

Never skip meals

Dieters make the mistake of believing that skipping meals will help them cut calories and lose weight. But when you skip a meal your system goes into starvation mode. Your metabolism slows down to conserve energy and your body prepares to store fat during your next meal. Additionally, going too many hours between meals means you'll be so hungry the next time you eat that you'll eat far too much. Don't confuse your body by skipping

> ### Did You Know?
> While you may have inherited your metabolism from Mom and Dad, it doesn't mean you can't do some things to give a slower metabolism a big boost. Increasing your muscle mass; eating high-protein, low-fat, low-calorie meals and snacks throughout the day; never skipping meals; and being physically active all speed it up naturally!

Drinking 5 cups of green tea may burn 70 to 80 extra calories a day.

meals; instead, eat small portions throughout the day. Try having three small meals and two or three healthy snacks throughout your day. This keeps your metabolism revved and working continuously and avoids blood sugar surges and crashes.

Eat small meals throughout the day

Increase your total calorie-burning capacity by having small, portion-controlled meals throughout the day. The act of eating helps increase your metabolism. The process of absorbing food requires energy. You burn calories with every meal as your body digests food. Keep your metabolism doing its job by spreading out large meals into smaller ones consumed throughout the day. You will end up burning more calories while still eating the same amount of food.

Eat enough!

Ensure that you are eating enough to keep your metabolism active. Many people mistakenly believe that if they reduce their caloric intake to a very low amount, such as 1,000 calories a day, they'll be able to lose weight more quickly. However, your body and organs, such as the heart, kidneys and liver, need a certain amount of calories simply to function, much less to get you through a day at work, playing with your kids, and exercising. If you're trying to subsist on carrots, lettuce and chicken soup, you'll be too exhausted to do much of anything but sit on the couch, and you'll never lose real weight. Find a healthy balance that lets you lose weight but provides enough energy as well.

Never go too long without eating

Waiting too long between meals can slow down the rate at which your body burns fat, as well as cause blood sugar dips that lead to overeating feeling sluggish. Instead, try eating every 3 or 4 hours and choose nutritious foods — light cheese and whole grain crackers, small salads, hummus and vegetables, peanut butter on whole wheat toast, baked fish and chicken — and you won't overindulge at any one meal. Keep healthy snacks handy for those days when you're away from your office or house and won't have time to fix something. You never want to go more than 4 hours without putting energizing food in your system.

Men should strive for 120 ounces of water and women should try and get 90 ounces. Increase your intake in high heat, high altitude, low humidity, or high activity level.

Drink coffee and green tea

Coffee can be a helpful diet tool as it suppresses hunger and kick-starts the metabolism. Research shows that green tea can actually help you burn fat and increase your metabolism. Green tea contains very special compounds called catechin polyphenols. These antioxidants help you drop pounds by increasing fat oxidation and thermogenesis, the process where your body temperature increases as a result of burning fat. Green tea can also prevent the storage of excess sugar and fat in the body. Another antioxidant, epigallocatechin gallate (EGCG) has been proven effective at regulating glucose levels which may help reduce your appetite. Drinking 5 cups of green tea may burn 70 to 80 extra calories a day.

Stay hydrated!

Maintaining hydration is crucial for weight loss. Water keeps your metabolism working hard, maintains digestion, improves muscle tone, and makes your stomach feel full. Try having a tall glass of water shortly before every meal. How much should you drink? You need to drink at least eight 8-ounce glasses a day. That's the minimum! Men should really strive for 120 ounces of water and women should try and get 90 ounces. If you think about it, it's really not a lot. Buy a regular 750-ml aluminum water bottle (available at any store from Target to Starbucks to your local gym) and fill it up three times and you've already had more than eight glasses. No matter what your ideal water consumption is, remember to increase water intake in conditions such as high heat, high altitude, low humidity, or high activity level. Water is necessary in order for metabolism to take place, so being properly hydrated helps your body turn food into the energy you need for work, family and exercise.

> ### Trim Up to 200 Calories!
> **Pass:** Grande vanilla latte, or
> **Swap:** Sashimi instead of sushi rolls

Eat spicy foods

Some research suggests that spicy foods, primarily red pepper, cayenne, and chili pepper, may help raise your metabolism. These foods may increase your calorie burning capacity for up to 2 to 3 hours after eating. The heat generated from capsaicin can increase your body temperature and temporarily raise your metabolic rate by around 8 percent. While studies need to prove whether or not this rate has a profound effect on weight loss, eating spicy foods may also help you lose weight by increasing feelings of satisfaction. The additional water needed to quench the heat from foods may also aid in feeling full when eating a spicy meal.

Add lean protein to your diet

Proteins are building blocks for your body. Unlike fat and carbohydrates, which are primarily sources of energy, proteins play an important role in the function and repair of body tissues. Proteins help build muscles and can increase your metabolic rate.

It takes more energy for your body to break down protein than it does carbohydrates or fat because of the increased "thermic" effect of digesting protein. In all, the energy it takes just to digest and absorb protein accounts for approximately 25 percent of the total calories protein contains. Ground turkey, skinless white meat poultry, as well as egg whites, fish, and legumes, are great sources of lean protein.

> The energy it takes to just digest and absorb protein accounts for approximately 25 percent of the total calories protein contains.

Eat "negative calorie" foods

Nutrient-rich, fiber-dense foods burn more calories than they contain. Even though fruits and vegetables have calories, they are referred to as "negative calorie" foods. Negative calorie foods usually contain high amounts of nutrients and fiber, and the high fiber content requires more energy to digest than the amount of calories in the food itself. Some negative calorie foods you can eat are asparagus, berries, broccoli, cucumbers, lettuce, grapefruit, oranges, melons, peaches, and plums.

> **"**When you come to the end of your rope,
> tie a knot and hang on. **"**
>
> ~ Franklin D. Roosevelt

Chapter 3

Secrets for Planning Ahead

Your life is packed with commitments that take time and energy, and this also makes it difficult to lose weight. If you are heading to an appointment around a mealtime, you will probably grab something prepackaged or from the drive-thru, rather than making something fresh and healthy. After a long workday, having pizza and breadsticks delivered to your house sounds much more appealing than cooking a nutritious meal. Or, you might skip out on going to the gym when a friend calls and wants to meet for dinner and drinks. Indeed, work, school, errands, family, friends, and other daily tasks constantly threaten to derail us from working out and eating right. Unless you specifically plan to build healthy habits into your daily life, the best-laid intentions will fall by the wayside. As long ago as 400 B.C., Chinese philosopher Confucius wrote, "When it is obvious that the goals cannot be reached, don't adjust the goals, adjust the action steps." The way you have been living, sacrificing your weight and health in favor of other commitments, is not working. It is critical for the success of this diet program that you don't leave healthy eating to chance. Develop a game plan for how to avoid pitfalls and stick to your healthy habits.

Planning ahead, in spite of a busy or stressful schedule, can make all the difference between losing 10 pounds in 2 weeks and not losing any weight. Determine ahead of time what you will eat at each meal. Build a repertoire of healthy recipes and stock basic ingredients so you'll never be left wondering what to eat. Be prepared with healthy snacks. Make a mental list of the fast-food items you can eat without blowing your calorie count. Treat plans to exercise as appointments that cannot be rescheduled.

Burning or saving an extra 500, 1,000 or 2,000 calories a day will be a challenge already, so you need to plan properly to make the best food and fitness choices you can. Use the following principles to create a successful game plan for cooking, dining out, creating a calorie budget, and more.

Make a list of all the healthy foods you enjoy

Facing the reality that you'll need to create a substantial calorie deficit each day for the next 2 weeks can be overwhelming and daunting. You may feel like there is nothing you can eat when you are trying to lose weight. Make grocery shopping and planning meals easier by writing a complete list of the healthy foods you enjoy. Once you write down all the foods you love that you can still include in your reduced-calorie diet, your options will seem a lot broader and more appealing. Consider low-fat and low-calorie dairy products, cereal, meat and seafood, soup and canned goods, frozen meals, salad dressings, snacks, beverages, treats, and more.

Plan your meals for the entire week

Don't wait until Monday evening when your stomach is growling to try and decide what to cook for dinner. Use your weekend to plan your menu for the following week. If you plan ahead on

Saturday or Sunday, you are already in the mindset to eat smart and lose weight. Also, you will be less likely to use the weekend as an excuse to overindulge. Take a look at your schedule for the week and decide on a variety of tasty and healthy meals, based on the amount of time you'll have to cook. Then, head to the store to purchase all the ingredients to prepare those meals. Make yourself a quick, healthy lunch option each morning before work — think salads with grilled chicken or salmon or soup and half a turkey sandwich with veggies. Preparing for the week ahead and making your own meals can save hundreds of calories per meal.

Know your "calorie budget" for each meal

Practice planning ahead by budgeting your calories at each meal. By writing everything you eat or drink in your journal in the back of this book, you will know how many calories you have saved and how many you have to spend on each meal to reach your intake goals. Consider any starters (soup or salad, perhaps), your main course, sides and beverages. For example, have water: zero calories. Cross "beverages" off your list. Have a small side salad to start. Calories: 150. Have a 250-calorie turkey sandwich, hold the mayo, and you're at 400 calories. Now let's say you had budgeted 500 calories for this meal. You could spend that last 100 calories on a cookie, which provides a few moments of enjoyment, or you could save those last 100 calories. If you make this same choice every day at every meal and you will see the difference on the scale and in the mirror at the end of the week — guaranteed.

> Unless you specifically plan to build healthy habits into your daily life, the best-laid intentions will fall by the wayside.

Have a game plan for dining out

A recent study showed that people consume 50 percent more

calories, fat, and sodium when they eat out. But just because you're trying to lose weight, doesn't mean you have to pass on dinner with friends — you just need to plan ahead so you don't overeat. According to Purdue University research, eating a pre-meal snack of a handful of peanuts about an hour before dinner will lead you to eat less total calories and fat during your main meal. Also, a broth-based soup or small side salad are good pre-meal choices. To eat less, anticipate what you're going to order, so your eyes don't get bigger than your stomach when you're sitting at the table with all your friends. Almost all restaurant menus are online now, and many also provide nutritional facts, so check ahead of time and decide what you're going to have. Consider ordering an appetizer, such as steamed mussels or a Caprese salad, as your meal. Restaurants are notorious for doubling and even tripling portion sizes, so truly, an appetizer or half-portion is probably all the food you need anyway.

Did You Know?

Research estimates that soft drinks make up between 5.5 and 7 percent of the calories in an American diet! If you haven't already, give up full-sugar soda immediately. However, simply drinking diet soda isn't enough of a weight-loss game plan. Be sure you're not ordering the fried chicken bucket just because you're enjoying a zero-calorie soda.

Start a recipe folder

When you're trying to decide what to cook, you need an array of healthy options right at your fingertips or you'll be tempted to call for take-out or pick up greasy fast-food. Start keeping a recipe folder. Go online and print out healthy recipes from sites like CookingLight.com or EatingWell.com. Or, buy magazines like *Real Simple* that offer fast, healthy recipes with complete calorie and fat information and fill your folder with tear-outs. Better still, contact friends and family who are in good shape and ask for their healthy, tried-and-true recipes. You could even start a healthy-recipe email chain that lots of people you know will benefit from.

After a meal, you could spend your last 100 calories on a cookie, which provides a few moments of enjoyment, or you could save those last 100 calories. Save them and you will see the difference on the scale at the end of the week — guaranteed.

Make a shopping list and stick to it

Focus on shopping for only the items you need to lose weight and stick to the list you made earlier in this chapter. Grocery stores stock the most tempting foods at eye level and in the center aisles. It's easy to get sidetracked if you let your eyes wander. It's also hard to resist a good bargain. Sale items can be difficult to pass up, so avoid the "endcaps" of store aisles, which offer low prices on processed items that have a high profit margin for the store, like donuts, sugary cereal, soda, chips and dip, and other unhealthy foods. You will be less susceptible to bright packaging, enticing deals, and other impulse items if you put on grocery shopping blinders and stick to your list.

Don't grocery shop when you're hungry

Stores use merchandising tricks such as smell, product placement, overall store layout, and sale items to get you to buy more. These ploys encourage you to shop longer and spend more money. You may end up buying more food than you need, especially if you are hungry. Stop by the grocery store after a meal when you won't be

**Trim Up to
200 Calories!**
Pass: Butter on movie
popcorn, or
Swap: Egg whites
instead of whole
eggs

as likely to stray from your shopping list. Or, drink a large glass of water. The feeling of fullness will make it easier to resist food. Another tip is to chew on a piece of peppermint gum while you shop. You will be less likely to try free samples.

Plan ahead for travel

If you travel often and will be spending a lot of time in airports and on planes in the next 2 weeks, you must have a strategy that enables you to still lose weight. In-flight snacks are typically chips and crackers, with 200 or more empty calories in each tiny package. Airport food is even worse — pre-made sandwiches, personal pizzas, burritos, and barbecue are common layover fare, so you're looking at up to 800 calories. Ward off extra calories by packing portable, healthy snacks in your carry-on when you are faced with layovers, long flights or possible delays. Raw, pre-cut veggies, an apple, dried fruits and nuts, and whole wheat crackers with natural peanut butter are easy-to-pack snacks. Or, make a sandwich (hold the mayo) that you wrap in tin foil and eat mid-flight. Other travelers will be jealous of your healthy, tasty meal!

Outsmart the minibar

A weary traveller can easily be tempted by the hotel minibar and its salty and sweet snacks that are just an arm's length away. Practice this celebrity trick and save hundreds of calories by calling your hotel ahead of time and asking that the minibar be locked up or emptied all together. It's too easy to give into temptation when you're on-the-go, so plan ahead for an out-of-town stay. Instead, bring healthy snacks with you or stop by a grocery store to stock up on smart options to keep in your room.

Keep meal replacement options in your car or desk

There are times when a fresh, home-cooked meal isn't an option, so have some meal replacement bars and shakes on hand. While they aren't a long-term meal substitute, they are certainly the better choice when you need nutrition in a hurry and your other choice is the drive-thru or vending machine. Stick to drinks and bars that provide a balanced 40/30/30 or 40/40/20 ratio of carbohydrates, fats, and proteins. Steer clear of bars with too many simple sugars, which add empty carbs and don't satiate you over an extended time period. Instead, look for a bar with more fiber, which will make you feel full longer. And stay away from anything that contains partially hydrogenated oils, which are a source of heart-clogging trans fats.

Cook and freeze meals for later

Don't wait until Monday evening when your stomach is growling to try and decide what to cook for dinner. Use your weekend to plan your menu for the following week.

While fresh is always better than frozen, many busy people enjoy the fact that frozen meals save them time. If you like the efficiency and convenience of frozen diet meals, try taking one evening or weekend afternoon to make a large batch of fresh food that can be divided into servings, frozen, and reheated later. Soup, chili, and vegetarian lasagna are just a few great options that can be made in healthy ways. Store each portion in an airtight container, freeze, and enjoy for up to three months. Having a frozen pre-portioned meal on hand at all times means you won't be tempted to go for fast-food when you're short on time.

" Live to the point of tears. **"**

~ Albert Camus

Chapter 4

Curbing
Your Appetite

Our need for food is first and foremost a biological need. Our body needs calories, fat, nutrients, vitamins, carbohydrates, water, and proteins to carry out complex biochemical reactions that allow us to grow, heal, and function. But of course, if eating were primarily about giving our bodies the energy they need to function, we would simply take a pill or gel that contained our daily nutritional values and call it a day. In reality, eating is a social activity often dictated by our desires for certain kinds of food.

This love of food, or what we call "appetite," however, causes us to eat when we are not hungry, to overeat because we like how a food tastes, to crave foods that are bad for us, and to substitute eating for other activities when we are bored or restless. Our love of eating causes us to forget the primary biological reasons we are supposed to eat. This, combined with technological advances in food preparation and preservation and a higher standard of living, provides us with a dizzying array of choices through which to satisfy our hungry stomachs.

Controlling your appetite is one of the most important parts of losing 10 pounds in 2 weeks. The best way to curb your appetite is to continually remind yourself that while eating is pleasurable, you should do so primarily because you have a physical need to eat. Food is fuel for your day, for exercise, for mental focus, and for your well-being.

Indulging in the bad foods you crave forms neuronal connections in the brain. When these pathways get constantly activated and reinforced you end up thinking about and craving those foods all the time.

The tips and secrets you learn in this chapter will help you determine what causes you to eat when you're not hungry, restrict your desire for food when your body does not really need it, stave off cravings for high-calorie foods, and eat less overall to lose weight.

Ask yourself, What type of hunger is this?

One key to losing weight is to identify your hunger and stop mindless snacking and eating. People may eat when they're not hungry or they overeat when they are extremely hungry and have low blood sugar. Sometimes people eat more in a social setting, surrounded by friends. Other times, they eat more sitting home alone, out of loneliness or boredom. One specific food may even trigger overeating. Since you cannot avoid food, you need to identify your hunger and find a way to address that need in the right way. Figure out if you are experiencing true physical hunger, low blood sugar hunger, cravings, comfort eating, or social hunger. Once you are honest with yourself about why you're eating, you can put down the chips and wait until you're experiencing true physical hunger to eat a full, healthy meal.

Know what foods trigger your appetite

Identify the foods that send your appetite out of control. These are foods that you find yourself compulsively overeating after one bite. Common trigger foods usually combine sugar and fat, or fat and salt. Binges are linked to the food itself; for example, if donuts are one of your trigger foods, a single bite can result in you eating 3 donuts, regardless of your hunger, situation, or emotional state. Until you are able to stop these impulses, you should avoid your trigger foods completely. Avoid even walking past the bakery section at the grocery store. Don't have a box of Girl Scout cookies at home if you know you won't stop with just one cookie. For now, skip the office happy hour if you know you'll be tempted to binge on salty bar food.

Recognize that seeing foods you crave makes you want them more

Your sense of sight is a key factor in controlling your appetite and losing weight. Research has shown that seeing and indulging in the bad foods you crave over and over forms neuronal connections in the brain. When these pathways get constantly activated and reinforced you end up thinking about and craving those foods all the time. When a person sees a food he or she likes, the brain becomes very active; on the flip side, brain waves show less activity when people look at foods they don't particularly like. Even a photo of a tasty dish can increase your appetite. Don't linger over menus with large images of high-calorie meals and don't even look over at the dessert tray. Don't let your gaze wander to other dinners when eating out. Simply recognizing that sight has a significant impact on your appetite will help you fight the temptation to eat when you are not hungry.

Steer clear of refined carbohydrates

Refined carbs are items made with sugars and white flour, such as white pasta, rice, bagels, donuts and muffins. Ever notice how your morning bagel actually makes you feel hungrier after you eat it? That's because the body processes refined carbs so quickly that your blood sugar surges and drops. When blood sugar levels drop, the body feels hungry. So, you've not only eaten a 450-calorie bagel with cream cheese, you're ready to eat again mid-morning. Stick to complex carbohydrates that are low in fat and provide healthy protein, such as oatmeal, whole grain rice, yams, beans and more. These foods slow the digestion process and the release of sugar into the bloodstream to keep levels stable and hunger at bay.

Did You Know?

You may have heard that red wine is high in healthy-giving antioxidants; however, don't use that as an excuse for drinking alcohol and derailing your weight loss. Red wine contains 120 calories a glass or more and alcohol is known to stoke the appetite. To benefit from antioxidants, try drinking green or black tea instead.

Alcohol may make you hungrier

A night of drinks and dinner may sound like a good time, but it's wreaking havoc on your weight loss. The first issue is that liquids don't satisfy you or fill you up. In fact, research has shown that alcohol not only decreases willpower, it whets the appetite and increases cravings for high-sodium, high-fat foods (consider traditional "bar food," which is things like onion rings, burgers, nachos, and hot wings). There can be as much as a 20 percent increase in calories consumed at a meal when alcohol was served beforehand. And with the calories from the alcohol added in, there is a 33 percent total increase in calories. Secondly, after a night of imbibing, the alcohol is what the body breaks down first, before other nutrients, slowing the fat-burning process. The bottom line is, don't drink and eat and you'll save hundreds of calories.

Slow down!

You eat quickly because of a hectic schedule, because you're on-the-go, or simply because you're a fast eater. However, studies show that people who eat quickly consistently overeat and tend to be more overweight than people who eat slowly. When you eat, your body releases hormones that indicate fullness and tell your brain that you are satisfied. It takes up to 20 minutes for this process to take be complete. During this time, it is very easy to stuff yourself with much more food than you really need if you're eating quickly. Use smaller utensils, take smaller bites, chew your food thoroughly, take a drink of water, and put your utensils down between bites. Try eating half of what's on your plate, wait 10 minutes, then have a few more bites if you're still hungry.

> The majority of what your brain perceives as taste is actually smell, so if you saturate your sense of smell with a strong odor, like mint, the smell of food will be less appealing.

Go minty after meals

Studies have shown that mint flavor and smell may suppress appetite for a short period of time, so brush your teeth or chew a piece of mint gum after meals. The majority of what your brain perceives as taste is actually smell, so if you saturate your sense of smell with a strong odor, like mint, the smell of food will be less appealing and you're less likely to eat more than you need.

> **Trim Up to 500 Calories!**
>
> **Pass:** Frozen margarita, or
> **Swap:** Yoplait Light Red Velvet Cake yogurt instead of the real thing!

In one study from Wheeling Jesuit University, 40 people sniffed peppermint every 2 hours for 5 days, then sniffed a placebo for the next 5 days. During the week they smelled the peppermint, they consumed 1,800 fewer calories. Also, if you are susceptible to nighttime snacking, brush your teeth early so you won't be tempted to snack after dinner. If you can, keep a travel-size toothbrush and toothpaste set with you in your car and at work.

Don't go cold turkey with cravings

Don't make your favorite foods off-limits, because you will immediately crave what you deny yourself. And succumbing to cravings leads to overeating. When you eat sweet, salty or high-calorie foods, your brain releases dopamine and other pleasure chemicals. When you deprive yourself of these foods, your body shifts into hedonism mode, demanding what makes it feel good. In addition, people have a tendency to want what they can't have, what is "forbidden." When you go cold turkey from your favorite foods, you dwell on thoughts of those more, until you give in to your craving and you binge. Instead, treat yourself but in a smart way. Eat pre-portioned amounts of the treats you crave, such as the 100-calorie packs of cookies, crackers and chips sold at all grocery stores. Everything from Reese's Peanut Butter Cups to Pringles now come in 100-calorie snack sizes. Allow yourself just one of these packages when the craving for something sweet or salty feels truly overwhelming.

Be the last person to start eating when dining out

People eat between 40 and 70 percent more food when eating in big groups. We tend to adopt the eating behaviors of the majority, no matter how unhealthy they may be. Be the last to start eating in groups in order to lose weight and keep calories down. Also, recognize that social interactions within groups of people tend to lengthen mealtimes. Longer mealtimes increase the likelihood that you will eat more. Don't feel the need to keep up with the table and match each bite of other people's food with your own.

A recent study showed that people consume 50 percent more calories, fat, and sodium when they eat out. Plan ahead so you don't overeat.

Mix up your routine

Altering your routine can help you avoid the triggers and temptations that cause hunger and overeating. If you typically meet a friend for drinks and appetizers after work on Fridays, this may be a routine that has to change. Interestingly enough, the sights and smells of these familiar places may be triggering your compulsion to eat and not the foods themselves. Meet your friend for coffee one morning instead and order a flavored coffee without milk for a zero-calorie drink. Or, if driving past your neighborhood taco shop every day makes your stomach grumble thinking about mega-calorie burritos, take a different route. You can easily save 500 or more calorie just by curbing that craving.

❝Always bear in mind that your own resolution to succeed is more important than any other. **❞**

~ Abraham Lincoln

Chapter 5

Controlling
Your Portions

A few years ago, the North American Association for the Study of Obesity performed a fascinating study on portion control and soup. Some of the 54 participants were given a regular bowl containing a regular portion of soup and asked to eat as much of it as they liked. Other participants, however, were given a self-refilling bowl of soup. Soup was automatically piped into the bottom of the bowl as the participants were eating, making it impossible for them to ever reach the bottom. Participants were not told that extra soup was being added to their portion, and the soup was piped in so slowly it was impossible for them to tell that soup was being added as they were eating it.

Researchers found that participants who ate from the self-refilling bowl ate a whopping 73 percent more than participants who ate from a normal bowl. Perhaps more astonishing was the fact that those who ate from the self-refilling bowls did not report feeling any more full than those who ate from the regular bowls. Furthermore, the study found that a person's weight did not affect whether they were likely to keep eating from the self-refilling bowls. Participants eating from the self-refilling bowls included overweight, normal weight, and underweight participants. Across the board, everyone ate more, no matter what their weight or mood.

Portion control is threefold: being aware and anticipating situations in which you may be served large portions, eating smaller portions, and feel satiated by smaller portions.

This study proved what most people have already come to realize: the size of your portion determines how much you will eat, regardless of how hungry you are.

Another interesting study of the factors that lead to over-consumption, published in the *Journal of Consumer Research* in 2008, found that a concept called "extremeness aversion" also contributes to bad portion control, overeating and obesity. Extremeness aversion is the tendency for individuals to avoid the smallest and largest sizes and order the middle size — no matter how large. According to Kathryn M. Sharpe, Richard Staelin and Joel Huber, authors of the study, this concept has gradually led retailers to offer larger and larger portions and consumers to choose larger and larger portions. You may have noticed that businesses like movie theaters and fast food restaurants have begun to inflate the sizes of highly caloric items like popcorn, fries and soft drinks. The study showed that if a fast-food restaurant originally offered 21-ounce, 16-ounce and 12-ounce options for soft drinks, most consumers would rule out the large and small sizes and choose the middle size, 16 ounces. However, when the restaurant eliminated the 12-ounce drink, consumers would choose the 21-ounce drink, because the 16-ounce drink they preferred earlier was now the smallest size, or the extreme, making it less desirable.

Additionally, studies have proven that people are terribly

inaccurate when it comes to eyeballing correct portions. A study referenced in the *Journal of Marketing Research* showed that consumers' perceptions of serving size are highly unreliable and can unknowingly vary as much as 20 percent. Another study showed that consumers vastly underestimate the caloric content of the foods they eat. In a recent study, researchers asked consumers to estimate the number of calories in different fast food meals. Most participants estimated 700 to 800 calories for these meals — about half of the actual amount.

Portion control is three-fold: being aware and anticipating situations in which you may be served large portions, eating smaller portions, and feel satiated by smaller portions. While this may not be easy at first, you will quickly learn that you can be perfectly happy with much less food than you have been eating. And it should be fairly easy to recognize the environments in which you are likely to overeat. For example, certain restaurants are well-known for serving outlandish portions — two and three times the amount you need to eat. Or you may be aware that visiting family means large meals with lots of food. Having a plan going into these situations can help you maintain proper portion control — and self-control.

Did You Know?

Don't fall into the trap of the "health halo," in which people consider foods labeled "organic," "fresh" or "low fat" to be healthier than regular products. In a Cornell University Food and Brand Lab study, subjects were given organic cookies and chips, some labeled "organic" and some not. The subjects who ate the snacks labeled "organic" estimated the cookies had 40 percent fewer calories and thus, ate more.

Use these tips and secrets to keep your portions reasonable and your weight loss on track. Controlling your portion sizes is one of the very best ways to build a substantial calorie deficit each day.

Know the correct serving size for your favorite foods

Do you know what a single serving is for your favorite foods, such as pasta, chicken, rice, oatmeal, fruit and more? The reality of dieting is that you *can* eat most of the foods you love if you exercise portion control. First, that means educating yourself about what one serving of your favorite foods really is!

Keep in mind that certain factors affect food portions, such as the individual's age, gender and activity level, but according to the USDA, one serving equals:

- 1 slice of whole grain bread
- 1/2 cup of cooked rice or pasta
- 1/2 cup of mashed potatoes
- 3-4 small crackers
- 1 small pancake or waffle
- 2 medium-sized cookies
- 1/2 cup cooked vegetables
- 1/2 cup tomato sauce
- 1 cup lettuce
- 1 small baked potato
- 1 medium apple
- 1/2 grapefruit or mango
- 1/2 cup berries
- 1/3 cup dried fruit or nuts
- 2 tbsp peanut butter
- 1 cup yogurt or milk
- 1 1/2 ounces of cheese

- 1/2 cup dry beans
- 1/2 cup tofu
- 1 chicken breast
- 1 medium pork chop
- 1/4 pound hamburger patty
- 1 tsp butter or margarine

A way to put your frozen dinners to work for weight loss is to save the empty containers, then wash them out and use them as a model for proper portion sizes the next time you cook.

Learn to eyeball portion sizes

No need for annoying measuring cups or a food scale — a handful here and a scoop there ... that looked like a tablespoon, right? Wrong. Research has shown that people can't eyeball portions without some practice. You won't always have a measuring cup on-hand, and who knows what an ounce of something looks like? Create a system in which you associate the size of a familiar object, like a golf ball or your fist, to serving sizes of your favorite foods. You need to learn how to associate common objects with the serving size of foods. After some time, you will be able to recognize correct portions just by how they fill up a plate, bowl or pan. Here is a list to help you get started, or come up with your own serving-size associations if you like:

- Vegetables or fruit: the size of your fist or a baseball
- Pasta: one handful
- Meat, fish, or poultry: a deck of cards or the size of your palm
- Snacks (chips, pretzels, etc): a cupped handful
- Apple: a baseball
- Potato: a computer mouse
- Bagel: a hockey puck
- Pancake: a CD
- Ice cream: a tennis ball
- Steamed rice: a cupcake wrapper
- Cheese: size of your whole thumb

- Dried fruit or nuts: a golf ball or an egg
- Cereal: a fist
- Dinner roll: a bar of soap
- Peanut butter: a ping pong ball
- Butter or margarine: a postage stamp
- Salad dressing: a ping pong ball

Create a harmony between carbs, protein & veggies

A simple way to stick with moderate portions is to figure out the proportions of protein, carbohydrates, and vegetables for your meal. Divide your plate into halves. Start out by filling the first half of your plate with non-starchy vegetables, such as a salad, green beans, or grilled tomatoes. Fill a quarter of your plate with protein. Choose from fish, poultry, or lean cuts of beef. The other quarter should be a starchy vegetable or grain like sweet potatoes. Now you can ensure your meal is nutritionally balanced and that you'll feel full and satisfied.

Create a system in which you associate the size of a familiar object, like a golf ball or your fist, to serving sizes of your favorite foods.

Order single items rather than combo or meal deals

Fast food restaurants lure customers with combo meals that include a variety of items at a low price. Avoid these marketing ploys no matter how great the value. The amount of calories in a combo meal can contain more than a days worth of calories. For example, a quarter-pound cheeseburger, large fries, and a 21-ounce milkshake has over 1,800 calories. If you have to eat fast-food, you can still lose weight by creating your own combo. Places like McDonald's will let you make substitutions, such as apple slices for fries and grilled chicken for breaded and fried chicken.

The kids' menu also often includes more reasonable portions.

Eat from smaller dishware and silverware

One trick that can help control portion size when you're eating at home is using smaller plates, bowls, glasses and silverware. Think about it: If you're using a large dinner plate, you're more inclined to fill it completely with spaghetti and meatballs — and eat the whole plate of food. But if you eat with smaller dishware, it gives the impression that there is more food or drink, so your brain will report that you're full and satisfied from a smaller portion. And using smaller spoons and forks means taking smaller bites, eating more slowly and enjoying your meal longer, giving your body time to feel satiated.

Order a "bistro size" or "lunch portion" of salads and entrées. This portion size will leave you happy and full at the majority of restaurants.

Stock your freezer with healthy frozen foods

If your freezer is full of healthy frozen entrees and frozen meats and vegetables, you won't be tempted to call for take-out or get fast-food when you're hungry. Stock up on meals with up to 400 calories and less than 10 grams of fat, as well as items such as frozen peas, broccoli, spinach, berries, boneless and skinless chicken breasts, fish, shrimp, pork loin, ground turkey, and more. On the other hand, items to leave out of your freezer include ice cream, chocolate, alcohol and any other temptations.

Use frozen diet dinner trays for portion control

An awesome benefit of frozen diet meals is that they are nutritionally balanced, portion-controlled and provide an accurate idea of how much fat, carbs, sodium and calories you're eating. Another way to put your frozen dinners to work for weight loss is to save a few of the empty containers when you're done eating. Wash them out and use them as a model for proper portion sizes the next time you cook. Frozen diet meals can be an excellent teacher for understanding the right ratios of protein to vegetables to starch to sauce.

Don't put serving dishes out on the table

Part of losing weight and exercising portion control is feeling satiated from a smaller amount of food than you're used to. It's important to know that sense of satiation is very visual. If you set bowls or pans of food out on the table, you are simply encouraging yourself to take seconds. Serve yourself a reasonable portion size while you're in the kitchen, then put the rest of the food away for leftovers. This way you won't be tempted to take more of anything. Savor and appreciate each bite. After you eat, busy yourself with dishes and cleaning up your cooking space — this gives your brain a chance to register that your body is full, and you won't feel the need to grab another dinner roll or helping of potatoes.

Take the food out of its container

When you're eating out of a container, there is also a tendency to feel like you haven't eaten enough to satisfy you. If you take the food out of the packaging your brain will register just how much you're really eating. A yogurt may not look like much in its packaging, but you'll discover its contents actually fill a bowl. And how many times have you gotten to the bottom of a 100-calorie snack pack and commented, "There were only four cookies in there!" If you pour them out ahead of time, your brain has a chance to register that you are, in fact, eating a full handful of small cookies, which is a healthy portion for losing weight.

Order the smallest size meal when dining out

We all know that portion control is much easier when we're eating at home. At home we can regulate how much we put on a plate, whereas at a restaurant, portions are often two and even three times the size of what we'd serve ourselves. A huge part of losing 10 pounds is learning to identify a smart portion when dining out. Always opt for the smallest portion size available. Many restaurants offer a "bistro size" or "lunch portion" of their salads and entrées. This portion size will leave you happy and full at 99 percent of restaurants. Or, order an appetizer version of a full entrée, such a veggie quesadilla or steamed mussels. When you find yourself wondering, "Will the half salad be enough?" remember that restaurants very often inflate portion sizes in order to charge more. Cut calories (and save money) by opting for the smaller portion.

Exercise nut portion control!

People who include nuts in their diet often have lower risk of heart disease; however, enjoy them in moderation, because nuts are very calorie-dense.

While studies have shown that people who include nuts in their diets often have lower risk of heart disease, nuts are also very calorie-dense, much of which is from fat. Nuts are only beneficial if they are eaten in careful moderation and do not significantly contribute to your daily calorie count. Unfortunately, because nuts come in large tins and bags, it is just too easy to snack on them by the handful and wreak havoc on your weight loss.

Know that not all nuts are created equal! Good nuts include almonds, walnuts, peanuts and pistachios. Not-so-good nuts, such as macadamias, pecans and Brazil nuts, are high in fat and calories. Because all nuts are calorie-dense, stick to about an ounce of nuts, which equals 160 to 200 calories.

NutHealth.org lists the following as the number of nuts per serving:

After you eat, busy yourself with dishes and cleaning up your cooking space — this gives your brain a chance to register that your body is full, and you won't feel the need to grab another dinner roll or helping of potatoes.

- Almonds: 20-24
- Cashews: 16-18
- Macadamias: 10-12
- Brazil nuts: 6-8
- Hazelnuts: 18-20
- Pecans: 18-20 halves
- Pistachios: 45-47
- Pine Nuts: 150-157
- Walnuts: 8-11 halves

Nuts make an easy, crunchy snack, just make sure you always count them out into snack-size baggies. Never try to ration while eating from a jar or bag of nuts — you'll surely overdo it. And be smart: Pass on anything honey-roasted, candied, oil-roasted, or covered in chocolate or yogurt. Raw, unsalted, unroasted nuts are the ones that will make you feel full and satisfied while keeping your calories down. In the right portions, they can be part of a successful weight-loss plan.

Ask for a doggie bag right away

Another smart dieters' trick is to ask for a doggie bag or to-go container as soon as your entrée touches down on the table. Determine an appropriate portion and set aside the rest for leftovers. When the entire meal stays on your plate, you are constantly tempted to keep eating and eating until your plate is bare. Think about how many times you've thought, *Well, I've eaten two-thirds of this meal already, so I may as well finish the rest.* Store half your meal out of sight and feel content when the plate is empty.

Split your meal in half

You can cut calories and still enjoy your favorite foods by dividing your meal and only eating half.

Extremeness aversion is the tendency to avoid the smallest and largest sizes and order the middle size — no matter how large. Be wary of this when you order items like movie theater popcorn and soda at fast-food restaurants, and always stick to the smallest size.

One way to do this is to split your meal with a friend. Or, if you and your dining companion can't agree, you can substitute the other half of your meal with a broth-based soup, fresh veggies, or a piece of fruit. For instance, instead of two slices of pepperoni pizza, replace the second piece of pizza with a garden salad and light dressing. This simple change can save you about 350 calories. Substitute water with lemon or sparkling water, like Perrier, instead of a soda and you've saved 500 calories right there.

" Divide each difficulty into as many parts as is feasible and necessary to resolve it. **"**

~ Rene Descartes

Chapter 6

Put an End to Mindless Eating

With our busy lives and schedules, so much of eating happens while we multitask or are on-the-go — at desks, in front of the TV, with friends, or in cars. Unfortunately, eating while distracted or while working on something else at the same time leads to overeating. Mindless eating is the downfall of many dieters. The hand-to-mouth action of eating can become addictive and, before you know it, you've gone through a large bag of chips or eaten an entire plate of fries that you didn't even order! Losing weight comes from holding yourself accountable — including your guilty pleasures, little indulgences and bad habits.

You must learn to pay attention while food is around you. One key is, of course, keeping a food diary, which is the single-best way to stay accountable for and aware of what you're eating. Stop functioning on auto-pilot and start paying attention to what you're eating, when you're eating, and where you're eating. Most environments offer cues and clues that you may be tempted to eat too much, and you must pay attention to those and get your willpower ready. You probably also harbor several unconscious habits that cause you to snack and eat without even realizing it. These are opportunities to change your behavior and cut hundreds of extra calories from your day!

Because food provides pleasure and comfort for so many people, and because calories sneak up on you in so many places, you must stop mindlessly eating in order to lose up to 10 pounds in 2 weeks. Wake up! Pay attention! Savor the healthy foods you eat but make eating an experience more about fueling your body than about enjoyment. Truly, the most wonderful feeling will be when you step on the scale at the end of each week and see the weight dropping off!

Just like the old adage, "Don't grocery shop while you're hungry," don't cook while you're starving either. Start making a meal before you're hungry so you don't snack while cooking.

Keep a food diary!

A hugely important step to eating fewer calories and burning through unwanted pounds is keeping a food diary. Keeping track of what you eat and drink keeps you accountable and aware and prevents mindless snacking. Luckily, this journal comes equipped with a 14-day food and fitness diary, but you'll want to keep maintaining one even after you've lost your 10 pounds. Why? For one, you probably have no idea how many calories or grams of fat are in much of what you eat. Research has shown again and again that people grossly underestimate the number of calories in their food — they are usually off by about 50 percent! Additionally, people tend to have generous and selective memories when it comes to what they have eaten. How many times have you "forgotten" about a half of a muffin, a handful of crackers, or finishing your child's cookie?

A study in the *American Journal of Preventive Medicine* followed

1,700 overweight or obese men and women (the average weight was 212 pounds) who were following an exercise and diet plan. The subjects who did not record what they ate lost 9 pounds. However, those who did keep a food journal lost twice as much weight, or an average of 18 pounds. So keep your food and fitness journal up-to-date and be accountable for every bite and sip!

Are you a snacking chef?

Are you constantly "taste testing" your chili every few minutes? Do you snack on shredded cheese while you're dicing taco toppings? Does licking the egg beaters after making a dessert date back to a childhood habit? What's the point of preparing a healthy meal for yourself or your family if you're snacking the whole time, adding hundreds of extra calories? Just like the old adage, "Don't grocery shop while you're hungry," don't cook while you're starving either. Start making a meal before you're hungry so the food is ready by the time you're eager to eat. If it's too late and you're already hungry, set aside a small plate of veggies, such as carrots or crunchy cucumber slices, to enjoy while you cook. A spoonful of peanut butter or a few crackers can also hold you over

> **Did You Know?**
> How many food-related choices do you think you make in a day? When a Cornell University team of researchers posed this question to participants, the average answer was 14. However, when the participants were asked to more closely consider a typical day, it showed that they actually made an average of 226 food decisions a day. One author of the study concluded: "... It is not unfair to say we often engage in mindless eating."

for a while so you aren't tempted to lick the bowl after making banana bread. Start paying attention when you cook and don't let hundreds of needless calories sneak in.

Beware of drive-by snacking

Food is often presented in a way that makes it seem casual, easy and friendly a bowl of M&M's on someone's desk at work, kiosks of samples at Costco, attractive hors d'oeuvres at a party, or a tray of bite-size tasters at the coffee shop. Without thinking, you grab a handful of candy each time you walk to your cubicle. At a party, you take something off every tray of hors d'oeuvres that comes around. As you chat with friends, "Ooh, I'll try that," becomes, "Sure, I'll have another." Soon you have a pile of cocktail napkins and crumbs in your hand. People often get the misperception that a few bites here and a few bites there are OK — but they add up quickly. You must eliminate drive-by snacking if you're going to cut out the hundreds of calories you need to reach your goal of 10 pounds in 2 weeks. Avoid opportunities for mindless snacking. Don't spend a long time chatting with a coworker who has candy or cookies at his or her desk, but if you must, be mindful of the presence of temptation and don't give in!

Look out for liquid calories!

Are you drinking your calories? Juice, smoothies, sweetened tea, sports drinks, energy drinks, protein shakes, and alcohol are all packed with calories, sugar and carbs, just like soda, and sometimes more so. Plus, have you ever looked closely at the labels of your Gatorade, Naked Juice, Arizona Iced Tea or Monster? Most bottled drinks contain more than 1 serving — 2.5 servings per bottle is typical. If you drink the whole bottle, which most people do, you're drinking 200 to 400 calories in just a few gulps. The real problem is that liquids don't fill you up, so you wind up eating on top of what you're drinking. Satiation comes from chewing, thus many times a liquid will be ingested unconsciously in just a few gulps, without helping you to feel full and without any thought for the calories you just consumed. It's easy to forget about 250 calories when they're in liquid form, but cutting out 250 calories can make a big difference in the amount of weight you lose. Drinks are a quick and easy place to cut extra calories to lose more weight.

Pay attention to environmental cues and clues that too much food is on its way. Family style serving dishes, carafes of soda or wine, buffet-style presentation, and oversized pasta and salad bowls are simply putting the temptation to grossly overeat in front of you.

Beware of bite-size

Unfortunately, our brains often trick us into thinking that eating something bite-size means it's better for us than eating the same food in its full size. But this is only true if you eat just a few bite-size pieces! And studies have shown that small treats, such as mini-cookies, actually lead people to eat more than they would if the cookies were full-size. If you wouldn't eat a whole cheese Danish, why eat four samples at the coffee shop? You're not doing your waistline any favors, and you're actually doing yourself a double disservice by pretending those calories don't count. Whenever samples of high-calorie treats are nearby, such as pastries at a coffee shop, remind yourself that even small bites add up to hundreds of calories.

Be the life of the party without overindulging

Always eat consciously. At a party, be wary of the hand-to-mouth motion while you're chatting with friends. You don't need to accept every time a waiter comes by offering hors d'oeuvre. Hors d'oeuvres are always rich and fatty in order to pack lots of flavor in a small bite.

Items like filled puff pastries, crab cakes, deviled eggs, bacon-wrapped shrimp, and creamy dips are popular and each has a ton of calories. You could be consuming 100 calories or more per bite! When you attend an event or party, stand away from the entrance to the kitchen so you're not the first guest servers with hot, fresh trays of hors d'oeuvres see. Also, a great calorie-saving trick for parties is to fill up lighter fare, such as crunchy crudités (raw veggies), shrimp cocktail, or smoked salmon, and allow yourself only one indulgent treat. Eat one bite to be sure it's truly delicious and worth the calories. If it's not, toss the rest away.

Trim Up to 300 Calories!
Pass: Cheese slices on sandwiches, or
Swap: Chocolate milk instead of a chocolate milkshake

Never eat in front of the TV

More than 66 percent of Americans report that they regularly watch TV while dining at home. Unfortunately, people who watch television while eating tend to overeat without being aware of it. Studies have shown that people can eat almost an entire extra meal's worth of calories on days when they eat in front of the TV. Television distracts you from responding naturally to your body's cues of hunger and fullness. Turning on the TV can trigger the desire to snack even if you are not hungry. You also tend to rely on external cues, such as the end of a show, rather than internal cues to stop eating. Keep the TV off and sit down at the table to savor the flavor, color, and texture of your food. You'll eat hundreds fewer calories than you would zoning out on the couch.

Keep food far from your bedside

Having food in bed is a habit that dates back to childhood for many people. You may have enjoyed a warm glass of milk in bed in order to have a better night of sleep. Maybe your mother brought you soup in bed when you weren't feeling well. Or perhaps the concept of "breakfast in bed" was seen as an indulgence meant for Dad on Father's Day. Whatever the case may be, know that eating in bed only promotes mindless eating. Bringing a bag of popcorn or a tub of ice cream into bed while you watch a movie or curl up with a book is simply setting the stage for overeating (not to mention making a mess!). Again, practice conscious eating by keeping food in the setting in which it belongs — at the dinner table.

A study in the journal Obesity reported that people consume an average of 236 more calories on Saturdays than on any other day of the week.

Look out for overeating cues

Environments that lead to overeating tend to give you cues and clues that too much food is on its way — now you just have to pay attention to them! Family style serving dishes, heaping bread baskets, short and wide drink glasses, carafes of soda or wine, buffet-style presentation, and oversized pasta and salad bowls are simply putting the temptation to grossly overeat in front of you. It's not just restaurants that are the culprit either; take a look around your own home for these items as well. Make your home less conducive to overeating and stay better aware of portion control.

In a portion of the Cornell Food and Brand Lab study "Mindless Eating: The 200 Daily Food Decisions We Overlook," researchers measured the amount eaten by 379 participants, half of whom were served with a particularly large bowl or plate of food. The participants given the extra-large servings ate an average of 31 percent more food than the participants with the normal-sized dinnerware. More interestingly, even when researchers later revealed to those participants that they had been given an extra-large portion, 21 percent denied having eaten more, 75 percent attributed it to other reasons (such as hunger), and only 4 percent attributed it to the environmental cue of the oversized plate or bowl. Researchers concluded that we are either unaware of how our environment influences eating decisions or we are unwilling to acknowledge it.

Hors d'oeuvres are always rich in order to pack flavor in a small bite. Items like filled puff pastries, crab cakes, deviled eggs, bacon-wrapped shrimp, and creamy dips can have 100 calories or more per bite!

Don't be one of the many people who is biased by the size of packaging, presentation, and plating. Look for common cues and clues and either stay away from environments that offer the temptation to overeat or be so conscious of the temptation that you monitor your intake carefully.

Make your own 100-calorie snack packs

Never snack on things like popcorn, nuts, dried fruit or crackers straight from the bag or package; you'll definitely overdo it. Bags and boxes of snack foods make it difficult to determine a proper portion size. Instead, make your own 100-calorie snack packs so you'll never be without a healthy, low-calorie snack. Put baby carrots, celery sticks, almonds, dried apricots, and whole wheat crackers into small baggies and have them in your purse, desk, backpack or wherever you'll need them.

While 100-calorie packs of treats, such as cookies, chips and candy, are now available, you should only purchase those tempting, sugary or salty snacks if you know you have the willpower to eat just one package. If chocolate chip cookies or potato chips are a trigger food for you, 100-calorie packs are just needless temptation.

Beware of Saturday diet sabotage

A study in the journal *Obesity* reported that people consume an average of 236 more calories on Saturdays than on any other day of the week. Theories on why? For one, your weekends aren't as structured as weekdays, where you have set times for lunch breaks, dinner, etc. Thus, people tend to eat carelessly and at odd times. Also, people tend to the view the weekend as time to relax and take a break from the routine of the workweek, thus, they tend to turn their backs on their diets and seriously overeat. However, losing up to 10 pounds in 2 weeks requires structure, and not just Monday through Friday. Don't let a lazy Saturday lead you to indulge in a calorie-rich meal. If you want to think of Saturday as a day to take it easy, use it as one of your days off from working out. But that's all the more reason to pass on a fatty meal!

TV can trigger the desire to snack, and you tend to rely on external cues, such as the end of a show, rather than internal cues to stop eating. Keep the TV off and sit down at the table to savor your food.

❝ Let us not be content to wait and see what will happen, but give us the determination to make the right things happen. **❞**

~ Horace Mann

Chapter 7

No More Emotional Eating

Ever heard of eating your feelings? Emotional eating is a huge problem for overweight people and in most failed diets, because the very nature of being overweight causes stress, anxiety, sadness and loneliness, which all contribute to the cycle of emotional eating. A study published in the journal *Obesity* reported that people who practice emotional eating have a much harder time losing weight, and those who do lose weight are more likely to regain it. The study concluded that, to be truly successful, weight-loss programs needed to teach their clients coping skills to replace emotional eating practices.

Emotional eating is simply a coping strategy. Anything from relationship problems to unemployment to depression to work-related stress can lead to emotional eating. Many times, emotional eating habits are ingrained and reinforced in us over the years, as we get older and the responsibilities and stresses increase with adulthood. And, unfortunately, emotional eaters are typically only interested in fatty or sugary snacks that completely derail their diet plans.

As this chapter reveals, positive emotions and people you love may be causing you to emotionally eat as well. You'll learn to recognize the triggers that lead you to overeat out of celebration, or the friends and loved ones who mean well but are actually wreaking havoc on your weight.

This chapter reveals fascinating facts about how eating in a social setting, with your significant other or family members, or around coworkers can determine how much and what you eat. You'll also learn about how your gender affects your calorie intake.

Because emotional eating habits are some of the most difficult to change (they often date back decades to childhood), these are also the behaviors that frustrate people and keep them from losing significant weight.

In reality, emotional eating revolves around having a very unhealthy relationship with food — using it as a coping mechanism, a comfort, a distraction from your problems, a means to fit in, or a reward. And when emotional eating spirals out of control, it becomes binge eating, the most common form of disordered eating, which affects approximately 2 million Americans, according to the National Institute of Mental Health. Binge eating disorder, like emotional eating, involves uncontrollable, excessive eating, followed by feelings of shame and guilt.

Whether you're overeating in a group of friends or pigging out on late-night junk food when you're home alone, you need to confront your bad habits and find better ways to cope with emotional changes and disruptions. Because emotional eating habits are some of the most difficult to change (they often date back decades to childhood), these are also the behaviors that frustrate people and keep them from losing significant weight.

Feeling powerless to food and your weight is a daily struggle. But learning the emotional triggers, people and situations that lead you to make unhealthy choices is the only way to break the nasty cycle of overeating that causes sadness and anxiety and, in turn, more overeating. Wouldn't you love to feel in control of your eating habits for once in your life? Wouldn't you love to find other, healthy ways to address stress, conflict, personal issues or to celebrate, without ruining your weight-loss efforts? Read on to figure out how to eat for nutrition and weight loss rather than feeding your feelings.

Recognize that emotional eating makes you feel worse

Emotional eating is a horrible cycle because it both stems from and creates feelings of sadness, stress and embarrassment. How many times have you heard someone say: "I eat because I'm sad, and then I'm sad because I'm fat"? People will binge on ice cream or alcohol when they feel sad, and then, in turn, feel much worse after realizing how many empty calories they just ingested. And the more overweight people get, the more they isolate themselves and soothe themselves with food.

> **Did You Know?**
> How common is emotional eating? Emotional eating may be a factor in as much as 75 percent of all overeating, according to the Department of Nutrition Therapy at the Cleveland Clinic.

As David L. Katz, M.D., a professor of public health and medicine at Yale University School of Medicine, says, "You can't make food the solution to every issue in your life and expect to be thin." Stop burying your thin, happy self under high-calorie meals! Your goal of losing up to 10 pounds in 2 weeks can be met with awareness, willpower and dedication. Once you realize how much better you feel from eating healthy and losing weight, you'll never want to fall into the cycle of emotional eating again.

Recognize these amazing differences between emotional hunger and physical hunger

You must learn the differences between and recognize the cues of emotional and physical hunger to find ways to deal with cravings and avoid overeating. There are several ways to tell whether what you're experiencing is true, internal hunger or whether your body and mind are responding to external emotions. Emotional hunger comes on suddenly, out of nowhere, and is associated with an event or emotion, such as having a fight with your spouse. Physical hunger is gradual; it comes on slowly and includes physical cues, such as a grumbling stomach, hunger pains, or slight fatigue. Emotional eating is typically for a specific food — chocolate or a cheeseburger — and needs to be satisfied immediately. Real, physical hunger can wait several minutes or even hours and a wide range of foods will satisfy it. Emotional hunger is not really related to fullness, so you may eat very quickly and won't stop eating when you feel full. You may also feel distracted and find that you eat a whole bag of chips or box of cookies without realizing it. Physical hunger, however, responds to fullness, and you will stop eating when you're satisfied. Likewise, you eat consciously and slowly, enjoying your food. Emotional hunger is coupled with feelings of guilt and shame for overeating, whereas physical hunger is not accompanied by negative feelings. With physical hunger, you recognize food as fuel and eating a necessary part of your day. Finally, emotional hunger may come on soon after you've already eaten. If you feel a craving coming on an hour or two after your last meal or snack, you can bet it's probably not true, physical hunger. With these differences in mind, you should be able to determine which type of hunger you're experiencing. If it's not physical hunger, focus on putting a stop to the craving instead of indulging it.

Head off emotional eating at the pass

Eating out of emotion is what is a called a "negative coping pattern," meaning that you are simply compounding your problems by being overweight. Awareness means stopping emotional eating before it starts. Figure out which types of bad feelings and situations lead you to eat out of emotion, rather than hunger. The five most typical emotions or states that cause overeating are loneliness, boredom, anger, stress, and fatigue. If your hand ends up in the bottom of the Snackwells after a fight with your sister, make a mental note of it. If your first reaction to an extra-stressful day at work is to stop for a cheeseburger and 6-pack of beer on the way home, be aware of that negative coping pattern. Then you will be able to anticipate and stop emotional eating down the road.

Emotional hunger is coupled with feelings of guilt and shame for overeating, whereas physical hunger is not accompanied by negative feelings. With physical hunger, you recognize food as fuel and eating a necessary part of your day.

Remove temptation!

It sounds basic, but if you don't have trigger foods around the house, you'll have fewer opportunities to overeat. You know the kinds of snacks and desserts you crave late at night, when you're watching a movie, or when you've had a bad day. Now, make a list of the things you can have instead — a 100-calorie serving of popcorn, raw veggies, a low-fat yogurt, or low-sugar cereal.

Find other outlets for celebration or comfort

You got fired, you got a promotion, you broke up with your boyfriend, your team won the Super Bowl — so you eat half a pizza. You tell yourself, "I deserve this." You use food to both celebrate and to help you lick your wounds. But what sense does it make to let circumstances largely out of your control so greatly affect your diet and weight? Why would you want the glow of new job to be outshined by the guilt you feel for eating a pound of Buffalo wings at your celebratory happy hour? Don't use food as comfort or celebration. Find other ways to give yourself a pat on the back or relieve anger and stress during a trying time. Had a great day? Go shopping and treat yourself to a new pair of shoes. Do something that makes you feel great, other than overindulging in food, like getting a massage. Had a crappy day? Need a shoulder to cry on? A burrito isn't going to provide the emotional support you need. Call a friend instead. Or sweat it out at the gym. Exercise is the number one stress reliever. And obviously, when you're exercising you're doing something beneficial for your body, as opposed to indulging in a calorie-packed meal.

Recognize if a friend or loved one is sabotaging your weight loss

While it is natural to expect that the ones who care for you would want to support you in your efforts to lose weight, many people find that certain friends and family members actually sabotage their weight loss — intentionally and unintentionally. Take a look at the person in question — typically, he or she is also struggling with weight, overeating and a sedentary lifestyle. Some people feel better about their unhealthy lifestyle choices when you live the same way. Many times, the person you are closest to has long been your partner in crime when it comes to unhealthy eating. He or she will feel isolated and jealous when you start making better food choices and pass on the beer-and-pizza-Saturdays that have become your tradition. Explain to this person that losing weight and keeping it off is going to require a complete lifestyle makeover, and you want and need his or her love and support to be successful.

While it is natural to expect that the ones who care for you would want to support you in your efforts to lose weight, many people find that certain friends and family members actually sabotage their weight loss — intentionally and unintentionally.

Stop the late-night snack attack

Dieticians and nutritionists commonly say that late-night eating is their clients' biggest problem that keeps them from losing weight. They eat smart all day only to fall victim to midnight munchies. Does that sound like you? Learn to ward of the late-night snack attack by determining why you're tempted to eat so late. There is an off-chance that you've restricted your calories so much throughout the day, and so you're actually hungry before bed. If so, try adding more fiber or protein to your dinner to feel fuller longer.

But truly, late-night snacking is just another form of emotional eating. Loneliness, boredom and stress are three of the most typical emotions that cause eating for reasons other than hunger, especially when you're home late at night. To avoid eating out of the desire for comfort or to relax, look for other things to fulfill this need, such as a bath or exchanging massages with your spouse. If you know you're going to be unwinding at home, find something to do with your hands other than eating, such as drinking a mug of tea. Warm liquids are also said to have a calming and de-stressing effect that helps get ready for a good night of sleep. Or, find an activity that includes both hands so you won't have one hand on your book and the other in a bag of Doritos. Type an email to a friend or knit. Cleaning can also be a good stress reliever that keeps you busy and out of the fridge. Whatever it takes, tell yourself you're done eating for the night after you have a healthy dinner.

Don't eat more in the company of others — male or female

A 2009 study in the journal *Appetite* studied the effects of eating in social settings on both men and women an discovered that women who ate in all female groups ate significantly more than if they ate alone, on a date, or in a group that included men. When men were at the table, the women ate about 450 calories each. By contrast, in an all-female group, the number rose to about 750 calories. Interestingly, while men were not affected by the gender of their company, they consumed more than 700 calories per meal regardless, which was higher than all the women in the study.

The five most typical emotions or states that cause overeating are loneliness, boredom, anger, stress, and fatigue.

The bottom line is, social environments lead to poor impulse control and overeating. Surely you've heard the phrase "Eat, drink and be merry." If your mindset is that eating out with friends is an indulgence or treat, you're more likely to indulge in high-calorie food, desserts and drinks. Both sexes should feel confident enough to say "No thanks" when a dinner companion suggests splitting the fried calamari or cheesecake. Alcohol and coffee drinks also rack up major calories, so order hot tea if everyone is having after-dinner drinks. Or suggest social activities that don't include eating! Do something exercise-related, such as arranging for a group bike ride, hike or entering a 5k with friends.

Maintain your willpower when eating with friends! A study showed that when men were at the table, a group of women ate about 450 calories each. By contrast, in an all-female group, the number rose to about 750 calories.

Know the few times when it's OK to give in

Certain holidays and special occasions, such as a birthday, Thanksgiving, family reunion, or New Year's Eve, mean you will want to indulge in a rich dessert, buttery mashed potatoes or a few glasses of champagne — and you have to know that it's OK to do so. Treating yourself, rarely and only when the occasion is particularly meaningful, shows a healthy and well-balanced approach to eating. You're not using to food to celebrate, per se, but you're enjoying a special moment with loved ones that includes a dietary indulgence. Just plan ahead. If you know you're going to spend a few hundred calories on these treats, you need to plan throughout the day and week to cut back in other areas.

Develop success from failures. Discouragement and failure are two of the surest stepping stones to success.

~ Dale Carnegie

Chapter 8

Choosing Healthy Alternatives

Americans tend to run in the other direction when they hear the word "healthy." Indeed, many people mistakenly believe that foods that are healthy are unsatisfying or taste bad. In a new *Journal of Consumer Research* study, researchers found that when people were asked to taste food described as "healthy," they reported being hungrier afterward than those who ate the same food when it was described as "tasty." In one portion of the study, some students were told they were sampling a new protein-, vitamin- and fiber-packed "health bar"; others were told it was a "chocolate bar that is very tasty and yummy with a chocolate-raspberry core." When they were later asked to rate their hunger, those who sampled the "health bar" rated themselves hungrier than those who ate the identical "tasty" bar. In a second portion of the study, participants were given a piece of bread either described as being "low-fat and nutritious" or "tasty, with a thick crust and soft center." After sampling the bread, participants were offered pretzels; those who ate the "healthy" bread ate more pretzels than those who sampled the "tasty" bread. This study showed that not only do people expect healthy food to be unsatisfying, it actually makes them hungrier than if they had eaten nothing at all. In the end, "healthy" foods made subjects eat in excess.

As a nation, we have been somewhat brainwashed to view reduced or low-fat foods as second-class to the original. But in many cases, reduced fat or low-cal foods are indistinguishable from their higher calorie counterparts. Sometimes, the low-fat version is actually tastier! To Lose up to 10 pounds in 2 weeks, you need to change your perception that healthy foods will not satisfy you as much as your favorite dishes. In fact, you will probably find that once you continuously substitute vegetables, fruits and whole grains for greasy, fried fast-food meals, you will start to prefer the fresh, clean taste of lower-calorie foods.

In order to lose weight, you must make healthy tradeoffs. Giving up desserts in favor of fruit, for instance, can help you drop unwanted pounds quickly. Or eating out less and cooking at home more — although eating out may be more fun — saves hundreds of calories at each meal. In weight loss, tradeoffs usually mean giving up something you enjoy for something less instantly gratifying but healthier in the long run. Diet tradeoffs are worth it because reaching an ideal weight, feeling great and being healthier are the ultimate payoffs.

Nothing will be more motivating than recognizing bad habits, beginning new ones, and seeing the unwanted pounds come off! Mark Twain once joked, "The only way to keep your health is to eat what you don't want, drink what you don't like, and do what you'd rather not." But this doesn't have to be true! Being healthy and losing 10 pounds is really all about making smart tradeoffs that have real benefits to you.

Modify recipes with healthy ingredient substitutions

There's no need to toss out your favorite recipes — just find healthy substitutions for the high-calorie ingredients. Your favorite dishes will retain their flavor and save you hundreds of calories. You won't even notice the difference! A favorite diet secret is substituting Greek or other non-fat yogurt for sour cream and mayo. You won't lose any of the creaminess but with zero grams of fat and packed with protein, you're making a smart tradeoff. Tofu is also good substitute for many ingredients because it is rich in high-quality protein and contains no cholesterol. Try using it in place of cream in sauces. Replace ground beef with lean ground chicken or turkey. If a vegetable recipe calls for butter or margarine, use chicken broth and herbs for flavor without the fat. Replace whole eggs with two egg whites and just a tiny bit of yolk. Use condensed skim milk for whole milk. Replace the sugar in baking recipes with the no-calorie sweetener Splenda.

Choose the right salad dressings

Salads can, of course, be one of your best weight-loss friends. Frequently eating green salads with raw veggies means your body will be getting crucial nutrients and antioxidants, such as vitamins A, C and E, folic acid, fiber, lycopene, and beta-carotene. However, to lose up to 10 pounds, you need to be consider the dressings you're choosing. A study of 1,000 people by Kraft Foods found that the top choices of salad dressing for women were Ranch, blue cheese and vinaigrette. Men's top choices were Ranch, blue cheese, and French/Catalina, and Thousand Island. Clearly, creamy dressings are the favorites of both men and women. They are also the quickest way to turn your healthy meal into salad sabotage. And, beware of vinaigrettes that load up with sugar to achieve better taste.

To save hundreds of calories and dozens of grams of fat, ask for oil and vinegar. A few splashes of red wine or balsamic vinegar are often all you need on a vegetable salad. Even better? Squeeze a fresh lemon over your salad for a zero-calorie dressing. If you can't live without your favorite dressings, many, such as Caesar and Raspberry Vinaigrette, come in a spray bottle version with only 1 calorie per spray (10 sprays are enough for a 1-cup salad). Don't turn your healthy salad into a 1,000-calorie nightmare; choose the right dressings.

Did You Know?
Data from the National Health and Nutrition Examination Survey compared fruit and vegetable intake to USDA recommendations. Shockingly, less than 1% of adolescents, about 2% of men, and only 3.5% of women met guidelines for both fruits and vegetables — despite counting foods like jelly and orange juice as fruit, and both French fries and ketchup as vegetables. Eat more fruits and veggies!

Cook veggies the right way!

Never cook vegetables with butter, excessive oil, cream or in the deep fryer. Instead, try a splash of lemon juice, a drizzle of balsamic vinegar or a twist of black pepper before oven-baking vegetables like cauliflower or sweet potatoes. Leave out the pads of butter from recipes like curried carrots — the rich spices already give the carrots a great flavor without the added calories and saturated fat. Experiment and you'll find that many vegetables, like tomatoes and bell peppers, are delicious when baked or blackened on a grill, without adding much of anything. Remember, the fewer ingredients the better when it comes to keeping vegetables low-fat and low-calorie.

Have whole fruits instead of juices

Whole fruits can help you lose weight because they contain essential phytonutrients and their fiber and water content help you feel satisfied. On the flip side, commercial fruit juice usually includes added sugars and 100 or more calories per glass. Also, when the pulp and skin of the fruit is removed, the sugar absorbs quickly within the body and can cause cravings later in the day. Juicing removes the bulk of the fruit so juice does not fill you up like the real fruit does. Half of a large grapefruit has 50 calories, 2 grams of fiber, and 11 grams of sugar while 8 fluid ounces of grapefruit juice contains about 100 calories and 22 grams of sugar. When you're craving something sweet and juicy, reach for the real piece of fruit rather than sugary juice. For a dessert substitute, try putting pineapple slices or halved peaches on the grill for a warm, sweet treat without high fructose corn syrup and added calories.

> To save hundreds of calories and dozens of grams of fat, ask for oil and vinegar. A few splashes of red wine or balsamic vinegar are often all you need on a vegetable salad. Even better? Squeeze a fresh lemon over your salad for a zero-calorie dressing.

Pass on ready-made grocery store salads

When you're cutting calories, pass on ready-made grocery store salads from the deli aisle. Typical choices — English pea, pasta, potato, Waldorf, macaroni, broccoli, chicken, tuna and egg salads — are all full of mayo. It's what holds these salads together, giving them their consistency. These are not healthy sides. These are not "salads" like you want them to be — "salads" meaning fresh, healthy and satisfying. A better choice that you can make on your own in a hurry: fruit salad. Chop a banana, apple and red grapes and add a can of drained mandarin oranges. Sprinkle cinnamon over the top and you have enough to feed two to four people a sweet side salad with no fat and only natural sugars. Another healthier, lighter option is to make tuna salad Mediterranean style, with chopped celery, olives, olive oil, lemon juice, and salt and pepper.

Enjoy a delicious bowl of soup

Warm liquids not only help calm and relax the body, they provide a sense of satiation because they must be ingested slowly. Thus, vegetable soup is a great weight-loss food. Soup is relatively low in calories per serving, and the high water content sends messages to your brain that you're full. You'll have to slow down while eating the hot soup and bites are always a spoonful. Have a tomato-based soup with high-fiber whole grains, beans, vegetables, and/or lean meat. If the bowl is small, pair it with a turkey sandwich on whole wheat bread (hold the mayo to eliminate extra calories). The extra ingredients will take time to digest and leave you feeling full longer. Avoid cream-based soups since they contain butter and fat and are high in calories.

Warm liquids not only help calm and relax the body, they provide a sense of satiation because they must be ingested slowly. Thus, vegetable soup is a great weight-loss food.

Incorporate veggies in unexpected ways

Not everyone who wants to lose weight also enjoys eating

vegetables. Even people who love veggies typically don't eat enough of them! Rather than sitting down with a pile of produce and forcing yourself to eat it, try sneaking vegetables into dishes you already love. You won't even notice they're there, and you'll be getting the nutrients and fiber you need to lose weight and stay healthy.

A favorite diet secret is substituting Greek or other non-fat yogurt for sour cream and mayo. You won't lose any of the creaminess but with zero grams of fat and packed with protein, you're making a smart tradeoff.

Some great ideas for incorporating vegetables in unexpected ways include pureeing carrots and zucchini in marinara sauce, meatballs, and burger patties; adding sweet potatoes to pancake batter; substituting baked butternut squash for pasta in mac 'n' cheese; and using steamed cauliflower in mashed potatoes. Vegetables are a crucial part of losing weight, because they are fiber-dense but low in calories, so they fill you up longer for fewer calories. Plus, veggies are packed with natural minerals and vitamins to ward off illness and disease. Just because you're a former steak-and-potatoes type or you're trying to cook for a family that refuses to eat their vegetables, doesn't mean you can't get the nutrients and fiber your body craves to lose weight.

Satisfy a sweet tooth with spices

There are many ways you can satisfy a sweet tooth without cookies, cakes, candy, or ice cream. The urge for something sweet can often be satisfied when you add spices to certain foods. Add the spices commonly found in desserts — vanilla, cinnamon, nutmeg, clove, ginger, and allspice — to other foods that are already naturally sweet, such as baked apples, pears, peaches and sweet potatoes. You can achieve the flavors and sweetness you crave from baked goods without all the extra sugar, fat, and calories.

Find a low-calorie alternative to your daily latte

Unless you specify, coffee drinks are made with 2% milk, which adds fat, calories and carbs to your beverage. Additionally, any sweetener, such as flavored syrups, caramel, or cocoa powder, add dozens of calories and carbs as well. And specialty drinks typically include whipped cream, chocolate shavings and other high-calorie toppings. Even if you opt for a light or "skinny" version of your favorite latte, you're looking at 200 calories.

If you can't live without coffee, the key to losing weight is to go as pared down as possible with your selections. Start with hot or iced Café Americano (aka, regular coffee). Sounds dull? It doesn't have to be! One or two pumps of sugar-free flavored syrup can jazz it up. A splash of nonfat milk is reasonable. Cinnamon is also a favorite coffee condiment of many dieters. It packs lots of flavor without the added sugar. Making this switch will let you start your day with under 25 calories per medium coffee, creating a 100-calorie-plus deficit, right from the start of your day.

All-natural peanut butter is a great food for losing weight because it maintains blood sugar levels and has fiber to keep you feeling full longer. Instead of a high-calorie muffin for breakfast, eat two tablespoons of peanut butter on whole wheat toast.

Don't dip into fat and calories

Dips are popular at barbecues, potlucks and housewarming parties, but most — spinach and artichoke, French onion, 7-layer bean dip — are jam-packed with fat and calories in every spoonful. Most of the most popular party dips are the creamy and cheesy versions, which have 200 calories or more per ¼-cup serving, more than 10 grams of fat, and include several grams of saturated fat.

If you're attending or hosting a party, skip the veggie tray from the grocery store, which almost always includes Ranch dressing. Buy veggies individually (usually cheaper than the pre-made tray anyhow), such as grape tomatoes, celery sticks, bell peppers, cauliflower and snap peas, and make your own healthy dip. A great one, even for the cooking-challenged, is hummus, which is just chickpeas, olive oil, tahini, lemon juice, garlic, and black and cayenne pepper blended to a smooth texture in a food processor. Or to make Mediterranean layered dip, a perfect substitute for high-calorie bean dip, you can stack low-fat Greek yogurt, kalamata olives, feta, tomatoes, red pepper, cucumbers, garlic and whatever else you like. Top it with chopped romaine lettuce and sprinkle paprika over the top for a healthy, hearty alternative.

A great weight-loss food? Protein-packed eggs. A study from the Pennington Biomedical Research Center showed that participants who ate two eggs for breakfast lost 65 percent more weight than participants who ate a bagel, even though the bagel and the eggs contained an equal number of calories.

Eat more natural peanut butter!

Natural peanut butter is a truly amazing diet food! It has heart-healthy monounsaturated fats and doesn't include the hydrogenated oils, sweeteners, and extra salt of other peanut butters. You'll notice the label on natural peanut butter includes only two ingredients: peanuts and salt. It's a great food for losing weight because it maintains blood sugar levels and has fiber to keep you feeling full longer. Instead of a high-calorie muffin for breakfast, eat two tablespoons of peanut butter on whole wheat toast. And peanut butter on a banana or apple is a great snack.

Although it might have as many calories as a bag of chips, not all calories are created equal. Peanut butter's fiber and healthy fats keep you full longer so you'll eat less throughout the day.

Don't mess up the most important meal of the day

Yes, you need to eat breakfast—but it's what you eat that is going to help you or keep you from losing 10 pounds. *Parade* magazine's annual report, "What America Really Eats," found that breakfast is actually becoming the highest calorie meal of the day for many people. That's because breakfast sandwiches and burritos — generally made with bacon, ham, cheese, fried potatoes and eggs made the top 10 on both men and women's lists of most-ordered menu items last year. Unfortunately, these items typically contain between 400 and 800 calories (not including the latte or orange juice you're probably washing them down with).

A better choice for weight loss? Protein-packed eggs. A study from the Pennington Biomedical Research Center showed that participants who ate two eggs for breakfast lost 65 percent more weight than participants who ate a bagel, even though the bagel and the eggs contained an equal number of calories. The egg-eaters also reported feeling more energetic than the participants who ate the bagels. Now, you do need some carbs, but make sure they're complex carbs such a whole wheat English muffin or oatmeal (without all the sugary toppings). Complex carbs make you feel full and burn directly into energy.

Beware of low-fat products

A report called "Can Low Fat Nutrition Labels Lead to Obesity," published in the *Journal of Marketing Research*, offered a dose of reality as to why so many people don't lose a single pound from eating low-fat or fat-free foods. The study found that both normal-weight and overweight participants ate more when presented with a low-fat option of a nutrient-poor and calorie-rich snack food. Additionally, they found that overweight participants were more inclined than normal-weight people to overindulge. Why? The study contends that low-fat food labels increase consumption because they decrease guilt and give the false perception that you can eat more of the item. And it seemed that this was particularly true for overweight subjects.

Don't love veggies? Try sneaking them into dishes you already love. You won't even notice they're there, and you'll be getting the nutrients and fiber you need to lose weight and stay healthy.

In a portion of this study, a university open house and two gallon-size bowls of M&M's were set out, one labeled "New Colors of Regular M&M's" and the other labeled "New 'Low Fat' M&M's" (although no such low fat product currently exists). As expected, participants ate more M&M's (28.4 percent more!) when they were labeled as low fat than when they were labeled as regular. Furthermore, overweight participants took 16 percent more M&M's than normal-weight participants. While all participants increased their consumption, overweight subjects ate an average of 90 additional calories more of the candies labeled as "low fat."

> **❝** Never go backward. Attempt, and do it with all your might. **❞**
>
> ~ Charles Simmons

Chapter 9

What to Do When Dining Out

A recent survey found that the majority of dieters said that dining out represented the biggest challenge to their weight loss. While able to stick to their eating plan at home, at work, and even at friends' houses, once in a restaurant, their goals and willpower quickly unraveled. Why does dining out present such a challenge to so many people? One reason is that restaurant food is cooked primarily with your palate in mind, not your waistline. Indeed, chefs go to great lengths to include sauces, batters, and other calorie-laden accessories to dishes to improve their flavor and presentation.

Because you cannot control the meal's ingredients, you may end up eating far more calories than you would like. Statistics show that people eat an average of 500 calories more when dining out than at home. For example, if you made yourself a hamburger at home, you might choose a low-fat burger, or maybe even substitute it with a turkey or veggie burger. You might choose a low-fat or multi-grain bun, skip the cheese, and serve it with a small side salad. But in a restaurant, you will be served a giant burger, up to a half-pound in size. The burger could be topped with special sauces, cheese, and bacon and served with potato salad or fries on the side. Once these items are in front of you, you will surely be tempted to eat them.

To compound the problem, restaurant portions in the U.S. have nearly tripled in size over the last few decades. Have you ever heard someone who traveled abroad complain about the small portion sizes in Europe? That's because in Italy, for example, meat, pasta and vegetables are ordered and served as individual courses, whereas Americans are used to having all three come piled high in the same dish. In the U.S., you're eating far more at a restaurant than you would if you were cooking for yourself at home. A recent study showed that people consume 50 percent more calories, fat and sodium when they eat out. Therefore, when dining out you must make an extra effort to control the ingredients and portion size of the meal you order the same way you would when cooking at home. Don't be embarrassed to inquire about how something is prepared or served and ask for substitutions if necessary. And you never need to feel like you have to eat everything on your plate. The "clean plate" rule of your childhood no longer needs to apply!

You never need to feel like you have to eat everything on your plate. The "clean plate" rule of your childhood no longer needs to apply!

Finally, as this chapter discusses, restaurant menus have been set up to make food sound as appealing as possible and many have photos, as well. The name of the Molten Chocolate Lava Cake with Crème Fraiche already sounds delicious, but when coupled with a photo, it's all you can do not to order one to enjoy all by yourself. And if the menu doesn't tempt you enough, the servers at restaurants have been coached to sell you certain dishes, drinks and desserts.

Luckily, American restaurants are finally beginning to accommodate the public's interest in losing weight. National chains and fast-food restaurants now offer healthy or low-calorie dishes that help the calorie-conscious have a pleasant dining experience. And as part of the 2010 national health care reform bill, any fast-food or chain restaurant with 20 or more locations will be required to post calorie counts right on menus, menu boards and even drive-thrus. The idea is that with the nutritional information right in front of you, clueless eaters and calorie-counters alike will be able to make smart choices that eliminate hundreds of calories.

Don't starve yourself all day before dining out

Don't make the common mistake of barely eating all day in anticipation of dinner with friends. You'll be starving come dinnertime and you'll overeat. Instead, eat normally throughout the day and have a small snack before you leave for your dinner. According to Purdue University

Did You Know?
Beware of your neighborhood chophouse! Most steak restaurants not only cook their steaks in butter, but they pour another 1/2 cup of butter over the meat at the last minute to give it that tableside sizzle. The next time you dine out, ask for your steak prepared without butter, and choose a lean cut of meat that is less than 6 ounces. Typically, anything labeled "loin" or "round" is lean. The seven leanest cuts of beef are eye round, top round, round tip, top sirloin, bottom round, top loin, and tenderloin.

research, eating a handful of peanuts about an hour before dinner will cause you to eat less total calories and fat during your main meal. Or, in case you don't have a chance to eat prior to your meal, order a broth-based soup or small side salad as a starter. Both contain about 150 calories, will fill you up, and lead you to eat less of your main meal.

Decide what to order ahead of time

Before you leave for a restaurant, check the online menu and decide on a few options that you can order and still work toward your target calorie deficit. Many locations now offer their nutritional facts online, but if your eatery doesn't, some safe bets are chicken, fish or lean steak with vegetables. Look out for creamy sauces and sugary marinades and glazes. If you decide ahead of time what you're going to order, you won't be easily swayed into sharing an appetizer or high-calorie entrée once you're surrounded by friends.

Say bye-bye to the bread basket

A fast place to eliminate 100 calories or more is to stay away from the bread basket when dining out. Although you might be able to resist the rolls through willpower alone, asking the waiter to remove the bread basket from the table is more foolproof. If you were trying to quit drinking, you'd stay away from bars, right? The same goes for losing weight. Carbohydrate addiction is a real problem for many struggling dieters, because eating carbs spikes insulin and lowers blood sugar, creating the desire for even more carbs. Don't put temptation in front of you! Have the bread basket removed or, if the people you are dining with want to keep the bread basket, ask that it be moved to the far end of the table, out of your immediate reach.

Beware of "healthy" restaurant menus

Meeting friends or coworkers at Chili's, Olive Garden or Cheesecake Factory seems like a good idea — large menus with something for everyone — but they're precarious spots for someone trying to cut calories. In an attempt to appeal to people watching their calories, many restaurants have started offering "healthy" menus — Applebee's has a 550-calorie-or-less menu, Cheesecake Factory's Weight Management selections all have 600 calories or less, and Macaroni Grill recently underwent a complete menu revamp that offers healthier choices. However, a 600-calorie lunch isn't the best fit for a low-calorie plan like this one. You want to aim for around 400 calories per main meal. Plus, these menus only really account for calories, so many of the items are super-high in fat, sugar and carbs. For example, the "Weight Management Asian Chicken Salad" from Cheesecake Factory contains 574 calories, 39 grams of fat, 68 grams of carbs, and 20 grams of sugar! You're better off sticking to meals with the fewest number of ingredients possible: grilled salmon (watch for any glazes and ask for it without them), brown rice, and steamed veggies, for instance.

Don't worry about what others think of what you order

When dining out, many people are so worried about what others are thinking that they order only a small side salad or whatever everyone at the table orders, only to overeat or binge on junk food later when they're alone. When they finally get to eat in the privacy

Before you leave for a restaurant, check the online menu and decide on a few options that you can order and still work toward your target calorie deficit. Don't wait until you arrive, when your eyes may be bigger than your stomach.

of their own homes, they feel relieved and comforted by the food.

Anxiety while dining out is most prevalent in women, who often worry about being judged for eating or not appearing "ladylike" to others. "When I eat in a group, I am convinced that everyone is thinking, 'Why is she eating so much? She doesn't need to eat that,'" said one woman who admits to this behavior. But you cannot let food control you! While it is important to exert self-control when you are eating in a group, don't let others' opinions or what they are eating affect you. Stick to your diet plan, don't give in to food peer pressure, and enjoy your meal. Your company won't be assessing what or how much you ate or didn't eat — they will appreciate that you have a healthy relationship with food.

Don't give in to eating peer pressure

You may feel like the relaxed, social atmosphere of going out to eat with friends makes it difficult to refuse a dessert or drink. You're afraid your friends will think you're not fun if you turn down food or alcohol. It's very true that social settings create peer pressure, even among friends. People who feel the need to eat to please others or fit in will always eat more in social situations. Instead, save hundreds of calories by saying a firm "No thanks" when your dinner companions suggest splitting an appetizer or dessert. Alcohol and coffee drinks also rack up major calories, so order hot tea if everyone is having after-dinner drinks. If someone questions you, just say you don't feel like drinking alcohol and leave it at that. Remind yourself that no one will remember who ate or didn't eat what an hour after the meal, so stick to your calorie budget for that meal and never feel pressured to overindulge.

Get out of the buffet line

Buffets are tempting because of the value, the wide selection of food, and the option to go for seconds. It can be extremely difficult to practice self-control while eating a single dish, let alone resist the wide array of food, drinks, and desserts presented at buffets! The standard buffet has over 100 different options. The uncontrolled variety at buffets and the mentality that you can eat as much as you want can derail the most disciplined eater. Avoid buffet restaurants, and if the place you're dining out offers a buffet special to accompany their menu, always opt to order from the menu.

Veggies on the side can't be buttered or fried

Just because you chose the side of vegetables over the side of French fries, don't pat yourself on the back quite yet. A side of vegetables is only the low-calorie option if you insist on having them prepared the right way. Unfortunately, the easiest way for restaurants to cook typical side-dish veggies like zucchini, carrots, and broccoli to taste great is to sauté them in butter and salt. It's a bad sign when vegetables come served on a small side plate — they're probably soaking in butter. The extra plate keeps the melted butter-runoff contained and separate from your main meal. Veggies bathed in butter or battered and fried mean hundreds of extra calories and tons of saturated fat.

To keep them healthy and delicious, ask for your veggies steamed, sautéed in a touch of olive oil, or roasted. Don't feel guilty about sending them back if they come prepared in an unhealthy way!

And when you cook them at home, try a splash of lemon juice, a drizzle of balsamic vinegar or a twist of black pepper before oven-baking vegetables like cauliflower or sweet potatoes.

Trim Up to 500 Calories!
Pass: 22 oz. fruit smoothie, or
Swap: Veggie lasagna for meat lasagna

Resist the sales pitch

Servers are trained to describe their dishes in very appealing terms. Plus, many restaurants offer employees bonuses if they sell non-entrée items such as dessert, appetizers, and specialty drinks. For example, instead of asking, "What would you like to drink?" they may say, "We have a frozen strawberry margarita that would be perfect with some chips and guacamole." Or, a server may bring by a dessert tray or drop off a dessert menu with tempting photos without even being asked. Restaurants know hunger is very visual, so seeing a slice of cake often translates into ordering it. Don't fall into this trap that ends up adding hundreds of extra calories to your day. Politely tell your sever that you are not interested in looking at the dessert menu and not to bring the dessert tray by. Stick to your game plan and order only the items that stay within your calorie budget.

Host your own dinner party

Enjoy the company of friends while eating healthy by hosting a dinner party where you cook a majority of the dishes and provide the beverages. Cooking at home means eating smaller portions and up to 50 percent fewer calories than you would at a restaurant, and you can control what goes into each dish. This is a big benefit when you consider that many restaurant meals are prepared with unhealthy oils, butter, and creamy sauces. Serve courses that include fruits, vegetables, lean meats and whole grains, such as recipes taken from Mediterranean cuisine. Serve natural sparkling water, like Perrier, with several choices of garnish to avoid the empty calories of alcohol. Guests can feel free to bring wine or beer, but you'll have an option for sticking to your weight-loss program. Organizing a group meal in your home means consuming hundreds of calories less than if you were heading out to a restaurant and you can still spend an evening socializing with friends.

Enjoy the company of friends while eating healthy by hosting a dinner party where you cook a majority of the dishes and provide the beverages. Organizing a group meal in your home means consuming hundreds of calories less than if you were heading out to a restaurant.

ff Success means having the courage, the determination, and the will to become the person you believe you were meant to be. **JJ**

~ George A. Sheehan

Chapter 10

Adopting Habits of Slim People

Do you have a friend who always passes on dessert, while you count down the minutes to treating yourself to a cookie or ice cream at the end of the day? What about someone in your family who loses 10 pounds without even trying, while you struggle with all your might just to lose a couple of pounds? It seems that all of us know at least one person who has an easy time losing weight, or even more infuriating, someone who is so naturally thin that he or she has never even had to think about it at all! Part of this person's easy relationship with their weight can be attributed to genes; indeed, some of us simply inherit high metabolic rates or extremely lean and muscular body types, which offer natural weight-loss advantages.

Yet naturally slender people also tend to have different lifestyles than do those who need to actively try to lose weight. They are less likely to use food as an emotional crutch or to resort to eating when bored, nervous, or tired. They are also more likely to be naturally drawn to physical activities that keep their metabolisms high and their muscles working. Most important, they tend to think differently about hunger, and thus make different choices when considering what foods to eat, when to eat them, and how much of them to eat.

What works for naturally thin people can also work for you as you continue to change your habits and lifestyle. Genetics do play a role; however, adopting the habits of thin, healthy individuals can help you to lose 10 pounds better and faster than you thought possible. Take the negative connotations away from the word "diet" and think of this program, instead, as mimicking the powerful and proven habits of slim, healthy people.

Never fall into the fad-diet trap, however. Celebrity or Hollywood diets, system cleanses, and outlandish weight-loss claims sound too good to be true — because they are. Fad diets aren't a lifestyle, they're a quick fix, and even then, many won't give you any results. And the ones that do aren't healthy. It isn't smart or wise to eat nothing but grapefruit or cereal for two meals of the day. You won't be getting the energy and nutrients you need, you'll feel sluggish, and you'll put the weight right back on when you're done with the fad diet. When you read health magazines, pay little attention to ads for fad diets or articles on celebrity weight loss and look for the "real reader success stories." These men and women have generally lost weight in a healthy way and have continued to keep it off. These are the diets and workout tips to model yourself after. These formerly overweight individuals have learned just what you will in this chapter: how to eat, exercise, and think like a thin person.

Choose being satisfied over being stuffed

Most people who are able to maintain their weight finish eating when they feel neither hungry nor full. Those who are overweight tend to continue eating past the point of comfort. The next time you eat, periodically stop and put down your utensils. Notice how your stomach feels. Can you stop eating now and feel satisfied? Find out if it is true hunger or habit that is driving you to finish your meal. If you are used to eating past the point of comfort, gradually cut back on portions and eat more slowly until you get used to stopping at a comfortable level.

Don't view hunger as good or bad

Hunger is just your body's natural signal to fuel itself. People tend to read into their hunger more than they need to. Thin people look at hunger as a simple signal from their bodies that they need food for energy. People who overeat and are overweight tend to either look forward to every meal, snack, and treat or completely dread every time they eat, fretting over every calorie. They consistently overeat or eat even when they don't have any physical signals to do so. Thin people recognize their hunger and understand where these sensations are coming from. If you find yourself eating for no reason, try skipping a snack. You may realize that you didn't even need it.

Eat more fruit

A study based on the nutritional habits of slim people showed that they have an additional serving of fruit, consume more fiber, and have less fat per day than people who are overweight. The additional serving of fruit may account for the difference in weight since fruit is naturally low-fat and high in fiber. Its bulk and

People who overeat tend to either look forward to every meal, snack, and treat or completely dread every time they eat, fretting over every calorie. They eat even when they don't have any physical signals to do so. Thin people look at food as fuel and recognize their hunger and understand where these sensations are coming from.

sweetness may satisfy lean people with a lot less calories than the cookies and pastries consumed by heavier individuals. Try to include at least 3 to 5 servings of fruit each day. Keep easy-to-eat fruits that are low on the glycemic index — meaning they cause the smallest changes to blood sugar and insulin levels — in visible places in your kitchen and office so they are handy for when you need a snack. Grapefruit, apples, cherries and pears are great choices.

Did You Know?
According to the Centers for Disease Control, leisure-time physical activity (gardening, walking, bike riding) has decreased since the late-1980s, around the same time group gym memberships exploded in popularity. Yet, despite 45.3 million gym memberships, national weight gain is on a steady rise. As may not come as a surprise, about 80 percent of gym memberships go unused. Recognize the fact that the gym may not be for you. If you're not using your pricey membership, cancel it and work on burning calories through recreational exercise instead.

Exercise an important muscle — your self control

One of the most significant behavioral indicators of weight is the amount of self-control a person has. Studies show that people who have fine-tuned their self-restraint have the lowest BMI. On the flip side, a low level of restraint has been linked to weight gain of up to 30 pounds. Your willpower is just like a muscle in that it gets stronger the more you use it! Learn to control your appetite. Plan ahead for situations where you have traditionally lacked self-control, such as celebrations and social events. Decide in advance what you will and will not eat. Pass on alcohol since it lowers inhibitions. You can't always control what is served; your willpower is sometimes all you've got.

Keep easy-to-eat fruits that are low on the glycemic index — meaning they cause the smallest changes to blood sugar and insulin levels — in visible places in your kitchen and office so they are handy for when you need a snack. Grapefruit, apples, cherries and pears are great choices.

Don't tempt yourself!

You're tying to burn or cut a significant number of calories a day to lose up to 10 pounds, thus, now is not the time to be testing your willpower. Don't tempt yourself by strolling through the frozen pizza section or chip and soda aisles at the grocery store. You know what your triggers are by now, be it baked goods or the grab-and-go candy bars at the supermarket checkout. Don't spend *any* time in those aisles. If you must be in the area, don't linger, and put your "bad-food blinders" on. Get what you need and move on. And don't push the limits by thinking you'll have just a few bites of birthday cake or just one or two cookies from a package. Eating the fatty, sugary foods you love sends pleasure signals to your brain and stopping at just a bite or two will be nearly impossible. Why take the risk?

Get moving!

Studies indicate that slim people move around several hours a week more than those who are overweight. This extra activity can account for an additional weight loss of 2 to 3 pounds! How much do you move around during the day? If you have a desk job, you might spend a large portion of your day sitting — although you don't have to. Get up and move around as much as you can. Walk around while talking on the phone; take the stairs up and down a few times; walk to the other side of the office to talk to a coworker in person, rather than sending an email. Your day should involve taking 10,000 steps a day. This type of activity is extremely valuable to your body's "non-exercise activity thermogenesis," or NEAT, which is the calorie burning process that happens naturally from everyday movements such as standing up, fidgeting, turning, bending and walking. A physically active person burns approximately 30 percent of their calories through daily "non-intentional exercise," versus 15 percent for sedentary people. Try to incorporate other physical activities into your day, such as vacuuming, shopping, or playing with your kids or dog.

Ask yourself, is it worth it?

Thin people evaluate what they eat based on how hard they will have to exercise to burn off the extra calories. If you are considering splurging on a piece of cheesecake, for instance, consider that you'll need to run for 45 minutes to get back to where your calorie count was prior to eating it. That's just to break even! And when you're looking to create a calorie deficit each day, you'll be way behind if you have that dessert. Ask yourself, do you want to negate a good, sweaty gym session with a few bites of food? Think thin and say no to any snack, drink, or treat that will mean extra hours of exercise (or depriving yourself of nutritious food) to compensate. In the end, you'll realize it just isn't worth it.

Get some ZZZZZs

Statistically, people who have less body fat get about 2 more hours of sleep a week versus those who are overweight. Researchers suggest that increased body weight from lack of sleep is linked to our hormones. Sleep deprivation decreases the amounts of leptin in our system, the hormone that suppresses hunger, and increases the levels of ghrelin, an appetite-boosting hormone. Cravings for salty and sugary foods increase and motivation to stay away from high-calorie foods decreases. Thin people tend to get between 7 and 9 hours of sleep a night. Give yourself the best shot at a great day of healthy eating by going to bed 15 to 30 minutes earlier than your typical bedtime. If you have trouble settling into bed, a warm bath or mug of non-caffeinated tea can help (warm liquids are soothing). Also, be sure to put away your electronics 30 minutes before you get into bed. Checking emails, browsing the Internet, and text messaging can make it hard to fall asleep.

> A physically active person burns approximately 30 percent of their calories through daily "non-intentional exercise," versus 15 percent for sedentary people.

Don't forget about your diet on the weekends

People who maintain their weight follow their diet game plan 7 days of the week. Saturdays and Sundays aren't free rein to forget about smart eating and overindulge. To lose significant weight each week, you need to resist lazy-weekend temptations: beer-soaked sporting events, late-night pizza binges, and calorie-packed pancake brunches. Too often you'll hear dieters call one day of the week their "cheat day," but consider that eating an extra 500 calories on Saturday may mean having to create a 2,000-calorie deficit on another day. It's just not smart or healthy. Maintaining similar eating patterns for all days of the week will help you establish healthy choices as long-term habits. Don't forget to plan your meals for the entire week ahead of time. This will keep you from wavering from your eating plan on the weekends.

Always ask for dressing on the side

As a rule of thumb: Don't ever trust restaurant salad dressings! Smart eaters know that even the light-sounding dressings on restaurant menus, such as raspberry vinaigrette or Asian sesame vinaigrette, for instance, are full of sugar. And restaurants are infamous for pouring on far too much dressing. A weight-loss tip: Dip your fork into the dressing cup several times and spread it over the salad. You'll get the flavor of the dressing without soaking your salad and adding tons of calories. And, if you don't douse your salad with a full cup of dressing, you can take part of it home to eat that night or the next day.

Thin people learn to tune out food advertisements and stick with their eating plans, no matter what special combo meal is now available. Be aware of how food ads affect you, and you'll be one step closer to thinking thin and putting an end to mindless snacking.

Tune out advertising

Online, on TV, or simply driving down the road, you are exposed to dozens of advertisements for food each day. An interesting study from the Rudd Center for Food Policy and Obesity at Yale showed that people are profoundly affected by food advertising and that these effects occur regardless of people's initial hunger. The study measured the amount of snack foods consumed during and after advertising exposure and found that both children and adults consumed significantly more of both healthy and unhealthy snack foods following exposure to snack food advertising. Additionally, food advertising increased consumption of all available foods, even foods that were not presented in the advertisements, contradicting food industry claims that advertising affects only brand preferences and not overall nutrition. Jennifer Harris, one of the authors of the study, concluded, "Food advertising triggers automatic eating, regardless of hunger, and is a significant contributor to the obesity epidemic."

Stay alert when food advertisements pop up around you. Thin people learn to tune them out and stick with their eating plans, no matter what special combo meal is now available at a neighborhood restaurant. Observe correlations between snacking and emotional hunger and advertisements. Be aware of how food ads affect you, and you'll be one step closer to thinking thin and putting an end to mindless snacking.

Practice positive visualization

Statistically, people who have less body fat get about 2 more hours of sleep a week versus those who are overweight.

Ask yourself, "What is stopping me from losing weight?" Do you believe you're doomed to fail? Do you start your diet imagining all the foods you'll miss or how hungry you'll surely be? Thin, healthy, fit people look at eating well and exercising as a lifestyle, not a punishment or a constant battle. Practice being positive about your new program from the get-go. Disassociate your eating plan with restriction and deprivation. Instead, view it as enjoying the right foods in the right amounts. Now, visualize your happier, healthier, thinner self after losing 10 pounds. Picture yourself in a swimsuit, lying in the warm sun on the beach, feeling confident. Visualize yourself cooking and enjoying a healthy dinner with friends or family. Imagine yourself walking into a party full of people and how they'll all notice your new body, confidence and happiness. You can literally feel how proud you will be. Positive visualization reinforces the reasons you're losing weight and keeps your eye on the prize.

❝ Plant your garden and decorate
your own soul, instead of waiting for
someone to bring you flowers. **❞**

~ Veronica A. Shoffstall

Chapter 11

Exercising to Lose Weight

Too many people falsely believe they can lose weight by simply eating less or eating better, without sweating one bit. However, creating a calorie deficit from your diet alone, without combining diet with exercise, is nearly impossible, if not dangerous. In addition, an extremely low-calorie diet means you'll lack the energy and stamina you need to get through your day. On the flip side, many people assume if they become moderately active they can lose weight without giving up their indulgences of ice cream, burritos and burgers. Unfortunately, neither is a healthy approach and neither will allow you to lose 10 pounds or reach your ideal weight.

Consider this: A University of Virginia study reported that to lose 1 pound of body fat you would have to do 250,000 sit-ups — or 100 sit-ups every day for 7 years. Exercise alone won't give you a flat stomach and defined abs — it's the layer of body fat covering your muscles that needs to be whittled away through eating low-fat, low-calorie foods and cardiovascular work that allows muscles to show.

Likewise, a Mayo Clinic report revealed the prevalence of "skinny overweight" people, or what is being called "normal weight obesity." As many as 30 million "thin" Americans are believed to have a body fat percentage that puts them in the overweight category and at risk for disease, despite appearing to be of a normal weight.

Healthy eating and exercise are a powerful fat- and disease-fighting combo and only with the combination of the two can you drop unwanted pounds and start feeling amazing.

Lose Up to 10 Pounds in 2 Weeks Pocket Guide covers the importance of redefining your food choices, creating a game plan to address each meal and craving, and making healthy changes to your habits. This knowledge will help you eat hundreds of calories less a day and shed unwanted pounds; however, you can't lose 10 pounds, and keep it off, without exercise. You need to stay full and satisfied throughout the day; cutting calories through diet restriction alone may very well mean you're eating too little, and eating too little leaves the door dangerously open for bingeing. However, including exercise in your weight-loss program means you can easily reach a substantial calorie deficit without starving yourself. Just an hour of exercise a day burns hundreds of calories, making meeting your goal very doable. In addition, you will find that exercise is energizing, builds muscle tone, curbs your appetite, and increases your metabolism.

Just an hour of exercise a day burns hundreds of calories, making meeting your goal very doable. In addition, you will find that exercise is energizing, builds muscle tone, curbs your appetite, and increases your metabolism.

So what is the best exercise regimen for you to embark on? The answer depends on your personality, interests, and individual abilities. You can do it all at one time or integrate it into two or three segments over the course of your day. Just be sure to build a plan that fits into your daily calendar and keep in mind that the common ingredient for any successful exercise program is to choose activities you will enjoy doing and that you may even look forward to each day.

Incorporate all three elements of fitness

Your fitness program should include all three essential elements for successful weight loss and maintenance: cardiovascular activities to burn calories, benefit your heart and reduce body fat; resistance or strength training for muscle tone; and a basic stretching routine to improve flexibility and prevent injury. Cardio is the most beneficial for weight loss and should be your main focus, but each element complements the others. Resistance and strength training will firm up muscles as the unwanted pounds melt away. Increased muscle mass will also burn extra calories throughout the day. Stretching and flexibility develop range of motion, increase muscle elasticity, achieve muscle balance, and protect the body from injury.

When you do cardio, you want to make sure you're moving continuously and getting your heart rate up. You should be breathing hard. The rule of thumb is, be working hard enough during cardio that you can answer questions but not carry on a conversation. Typical activities include jogging/running, elliptical training, bicycling/spinning, and cardio classes such as step aerobics, kickboxing, and aerobic dance. For strength training, aim for at least two 30-minute sessions per week that may include free weights, weight machines, resistance equipment, muscular endurance training, and toning activities such as Power yoga or Pilates. Focus on activities that exercise each of the major muscle groups or work more than one muscle group at the same time. Stretching is important before, during and after a workout. A study found that regular stretching can increase your strength by up to 19 percent when interspersed between weight-training exercises, for instance. Try doing 10 or 15 minutes of basic Ashtanga yoga poses.

Create a realistic schedule you can stick to

Schedule your workouts at the beginning of the week, just like you are doing with your meals for the week. Be realistic! If you're not a morning person, don't schedule 6 a.m. runs. If you like to relax after work, don't pretend you're going to take a yoga class in the evenings. Take a look at your calendar and pencil in workouts for at least 5 days of the week, on days and times that are most doable. For instance, plan morning workouts for the days when you'll want to meet friends after work, or schedule a lunchtime hike for a day when you want to sleep in. Building exercise around your personal schedule and lifestyle means you're more likely to meet your goals.

Look at your weekly schedule and be realistic! If you're not a morning person, don't schedule 6 a.m. runs. If you like to relax after work, don't pretend you're going to take a yoga class in the evenings.

Get a walking workout

Many people starting out a fitness plan turn to good old-fashioned walking. On a nice day, consider a stroll around your neighborhood. In cold or rainy weather, go to the mall and log miles while you window shop. Walking is a cost-effective activity that simply requires a good pair of shoes. Walking may sound too good to be true, but it is an aerobic activity that burns calories. Consider the fact that for a 150-pound person, walking at 2 mph, which is approximately a 30-minute mile, burns 189 calories per hour. Walking a 20-minute mile at a 3 mph pace uses 300 calories per hour. Walking a moderate, 15-minute mile, for an average of 4 mph, burns 300 calories per hour. The faster you walk, the more calories you will burn.

If you're not sure how far a mile is in your neighborhood, you can drive your car while looking at your odometer or buy a small pedometer to count your steps. The U.S. Surgeon General has recommended walking 30 minutes daily to strive toward a weekly goal of 10,000 steps, or roughly 5 miles. Those on a weight-loss program should strive for a minimum of 12,000 to 15,000 steps, which should take about 45 minutes per day.

Fend off food cravings with exercise

To increase your daily exercise and stave off cravings and hunger pangs, go for a walk the next time you feel like eating when it's not a snack or meal time. People often snack when they need a break from work or family, or when they're bored. Instead, try going for a 15-minute walk and allowing the craving to pass. Walking for 15 minutes will burn 75 calories for a 150-pound person. So, instead of eating a 150-calorie snack out of boredom, you'll have actually burned calories!

Did You Know?
One of the best predictors of maintaining a fitness program over time is exercising in a social environment, like a gym or fitness class, or having a workout buddy. Think about it: The people you see each time you exercise become friends and acquaintances who expect to say hello to you, so you're less likely to skip a class or workout. Plus, you're making new friends while you slim down!

Find solutions to your exercise excuses

There are many excuses to skip exercise or to let a fitness plan fall by the wayside after a short time. But you won't be able to lose weight without exercise to complement a reduced-calorie diet. Get out a piece of paper and write down the reasons you've been avoiding exercise, joining a gym, or taking a fitness class. Some of the most common reasons people use to avoid physical activity include:

"I don't have the time."
"I'm too tired and I don't feel like it."
"I'm not very good at exercising."
"It's not convenient to get to my workout place."
"I'm afraid and embarrassed."
"It's too expensive to join a gym."

Now write down solutions to these excuses. For example, if your number one reason for skipping exercise is "I don't have time," use half your lunch break to go for a brisk walk or take a bike ride with your family instead of seeing a movie (you'll still spend time together, get to interact, and do something good for everyone's health). The bottom line is, there is never a good excuse to be sedentary. There are great gyms and fitness facilities of all types and price ranges. If you find the traditional gym environment isn't for you, try a cycling club or dance class. If money is a concern, sign up for a hiking club — things like hiking, swimming, and rollerblading are always free. There are hundreds of ways

The best way to see your progress and maintain motivation is keeping track of the days you exercise in the 2-week journal in the back of this book. Seeing the days accumulate on your calendar will really keep you motivated for the times when the gym sounds less than tempting.

to burn calories, so stop making excuses — make time and find something you like to do.

Take measures to avoid injury

Nothing puts a cramp in your weight loss like an injury. And if it's something serious enough, it can even mean the end of your exercise plan all together. There are several ways to avoid injury when you're embarking on a new fitness plan. Always warm up and cool down for at least 5 to 10 minutes, before and after workouts. Warm up is especially important if you're doing early morning cardio because your body will be completely cold — like giving a car a chance to warm up after it's been sitting in a garage overnight. Also, give your body time to rest in between workouts. Get in a few hard workouts but then take one day off completely each week. For strength training, take at least one day off between sessions that work the same muscle group so you give the muscle fibers time to heal and strengthen. Finally, be sure you ask a trainer the proper form and technique for exercises and machines that are new to you to avoid pulling or straining a muscle.

Use your fitness journal!

In order to lose real weight, you need to expend more calories per day more than you eat. Therefore, exercise must become a part of your daily and weekly routine. The best way to see your progress and maintain motivation

Consider a virtual trainer — a real person who will create a fitness plan specifically for you, based on your goals and the equipment you have available to you. You'll get online tutorials, text message reminders, and email check-ins from your trainer.

is keeping track of the days you exercise in the 2-week journal in the back of this book. Seeing the days accumulate on your calendar will really keep you motivated for the times when the gym sounds less than tempting. Write down the activity you did, the duration of time, reps, and the intensity (or weight, if strength training). Keep track of everything you do, and don't underestimate what may seem like a smaller activity, such as walking your dog. Consider that a 150-pound person will burn 100 calories from just a 20-minute walk at a moderate pace. Every little bit counts, just like with calories, so write it down and applaud yourself for making time throughout the day to get moving.

Join an online weight-loss community

Create a profile page at an online weight-loss and fitness community and you'll have instant access to a huge group of people with similar goals, questions, obstacles, and tips for success. Seeing what works for others gives you motivation, and hearing about the ups and downs of exercise and losing weight from real people provides comfort and a sense of solidarity.

Enlist a virtual trainer

Hiring a personal trainer can be a great motivator and learning experience but not everyone is ready for the time or money commitment it requires. A terrific option is a virtual trainer. A real person will create a fitness plan specifically for you, based on your goals and the equipment you have available to you. You'll get online tutorials on the proper form for exercises, worksheets for tracking progress, and accountability in the form of reminders and check-ins from your virtual trainer.

Never give up!

"Don't give up, don't ever give up," legendary college basketball coach Jim Valvano told the crowd at the 1993 ESPY Awards, a night to celebrate the accomplishments of the greatest athletes in the world. Inspired by Valvano's fight against bone cancer, the athletes in the room also knew plenty about the resilience it takes to stay in top shape and perform under the most pressure imaginable. Valvano's words should inspire you, too!

Losing weight is a journey that takes determination and resilience, and exercise can be struggle if you haven't always been active. If you have had a busy day of work or family, it is tempting to spend an evening on the couch instead of going for a run or bike ride. One of the toughest things is getting back on an exercise schedule after you've missed a few days. But don't decide you've failed. If you skip a day of your workout, tell yourself you'll start again tomorrow. If you overindulge at a meal, be firm that you will have a longer, tougher workout the next day. If you feel like skipping the gym, tell yourself you'll do 30 minutes (odds are, you'll stay longer). Don't give up!

ff Without discipline, there's no life at all. **JJ**

~ Katharine Hepburn

Chapter 12

Maximizing Your Workouts

To lose up to 10 pounds in a short amount of time you need to make the most of every workout or physical activity you do. You don't want to do the same exercises or routine every day for 2 weeks. To optimize the amount of calories and body fat you burn during each workout and lose as much weight as you can, use the tips and tricks in this chapter to learn when and how to work out, how to dress for your chosen activity, and how to stay motivated on days when you're feeling sluggish or lazy.

There is a lot to learn and remember when starting an intense fitness program like this one. In this chapter, you'll learn the right amount of weight you should be lifting during strength training, how to calculate your maximum and target heart rates, find how much water you should be drinking, and determine the best time to get new shoes and which type to buy.

Use the tips, formulas, and principles of fitness in this chapter to maximize your workout results. Nothing will make you feel better or more excited to maintain your program. With 2 weeks to go to lose up to 10 pounds, you have no time to waste!

During a pre-breakfast morning workout, the body will burn more fat. You'll also have what is called the "afterburn" effect, which means that metabolism stays elevated for several hours even after your workout.

Work the "afterburn"

Do cardiovascular exercise first thing in the morning! During the night, your body becomes depleted of your primary energy source, carbohydrates. With that in short supply, your body begins to work from its secondary source, which is body fat. During a pre-breakfast morning workout, the body will burn more fat. You'll also have what is called the "afterburn" effect, which means that metabolism stays elevated for several hours even after your workout. Finally, working out in the morning gives you an endorphin rush and energy boost. This natural high can last for hours — even better than coffee!

Lift the right amount of weight

Building muscle helps you lose fat and drop unwanted pounds, but do you know how much is the right amount of weight to lift during strength training? If you lift weights that are too light, you won't see improvements in strength or muscle tone. If you lift weights that are too heavy, you'll compromise form and risk getting injured. You want to be able to perform 8 to 12 repetitions per set, choosing weights heavy enough that you struggle through your final few reps, but not so heavy that you sacrifice form. You should be maxed out by the last rep; if you feel like you could do another, increase the weight by 5 to 10 percent.

Another way to determine the weight you should be lifting is to find your "1 rep max" for an exercise (the weight at which you can only do one rep), then lift 60 to 80 percent of that amount.

Know how and when to eat to maximize your workouts

It's important to know which foods to eat before and after you exercise. Carbs that are low in fat give you the energy you need to have a great workout. Protein helps with muscle repair and growth. Fat also acts as fuel for workouts, although you should eat mostly unsaturated fats, such as those from nuts, avocados and fish.

Give yourself plenty of time for your body to digest a meal before working out, and specifically avoid fatty foods before exercising. Fats remain in your stomach longer, causing you to feel uncomfortable. However, having low blood sugar before a workout can cause dizziness and lethargy, so if you're famished, a small snack of peanut butter or low-fat cheese on whole wheat crackers can give you the boost you need to make it through an exercise session. After your workout, eating a meal packed with protein and carbohydrates within 2 hours can help replace energy-fueling glycogen stores.

Include interval training to torch calories and body fat

Your mission is to reduce your caloric intake or burn more calories through exercise than you take in a day. Interval training is a great way to blast through calories and body fat because it combines short bursts of intense activity with periods of lighter activity. As your cardiovascular fitness improves, you'll be able to go longer and up the intensity of the more difficult portions, helping you burn even more calories.

Here is one interval training workout that burns 500 or more calories in an hour. As your level of fitness improves, you should aim for a sprinting pace of at least 7.5 mph, a running pace of at least 6.0 mph, and a jogging pace of at least 5.0 mph. Your warm up and cool down paces can be slightly slower than a jog.

0:00–10:00 Warm up jog
10:00–10:20 Sprint
10:20–11:20 Jog
11:20–14:00 Repeat minutes 10:00–11:20 twice
14:00–17:00 Jog
17:00–27:00 Run
27:00–31:00 Jog
31:00–35:00 Run
35:00–39:00 Jog
39:00–55:00 Repeat minutes 31:00–39:00 twice
55:00–60:00 Gradually slow pace to jog/walk to cool down

Wear the right shoes

Just like getting new exercise clothes, having the right shoes improves your workout. Wearing the appropriate shoes for the activity — from running to weight lifting to basketball — also protects you from soreness and injury. For instance, running shoes are designed for forward heel-to-toe motion and do not provide the right ankle support for the side-to-side motion of activities like kickboxing or step aerobics. And not all running shoes provide the same cushioning and support. For instance, depending on whether you supinate (run on the outside of your feet) or overpronate (your feet roll inward as you run), you will need different types of running shoes. If you check out your old shoes, you should be able to see where the heel is worn down. Or, visit a specialty store to have your foot measured and your shoes professionally fit. A shoe should be snug but not be so tight that it puts pressure on the top of your foot or crushes your toes. And be sure to replace shoes every 300 to 500 miles, which you can monitor in your fitness journal.

> Wearing the appropriate shoes for the activity you choose — from running to weight lifting to basketball — protects you from soreness and injury.

Stay hydrated

Proper hydration is one of the easiest and most effective ways of boosting workout performance. Water is necessary in order for metabolism to take place, so being properly hydrated helps your body turn food into the energy you need for exercising. Water also helps your body regulate its temperature through sweating. Because vigorous exercise causes you to lose large amounts of water through sweating, it is important to drink water before, during, and after each workout session. Drink between 8 and 16 ounces of water in the hour prior to working out. Replenish fluids by drinking 4 to 8 ounces of water every 15 minutes during your workout. During vigorous cardiovascular training, or if you're exercising in hot temperatures, increase your water consumption in order to replace water lost from sweating. Then, drink between

8 and 16 ounces of water within 30 minutes of completing your exercise routine. Your muscles need water in order to recover from the stress of a workout. Drinking the right amounts of water after your workout will help reduce muscle soreness and help you feel less tired.

Build one or two "light days" into your weekly workout schedule, but make them count! Light days might include biking, walking, dynamic stretching (walking lunges, trunk twists or arm circles, for instance), and swimming.

Hydrate right!

It's extremely important to stay fully hydrated before, during and after your workout — just don't reach for a sports drink that is full of unwanted calories. While slews of TV commercials featuring famous pro athletes lead you to believe that sports drinks like Gatorade and Vitamin Water help you stay fit and healthy, these drinks actually contain up to 200 calories and 35 grams of carbs per bottle. The promise that these drinks will give you the energy and electrolytes you need to have a great workout is really just a marketing ploy. For instance, Gatorade was originally developed to help college football players avoid dehydration and cramping during a rigorous training program in the humid summer months. A normal person like you, who is exercising at a much more moderate level, has no need for the carbs and calories in a sports drink. Water is always your best option. If you like the flavoring in sports drinks, try a low- or no-calorie version, like Powerade Zero or Gatorade's G2.

Don't overtrain

Want in on a fitness secret? There is such a thing as too much exercise. Let's say you're preparing to run a 5k race, and you start running several miles every day. You'll quickly notice that after a couple of weeks of training hard daily, your body begins to feel fatigued more quickly. Your muscles ache and you feel tired after just a short distance. You may find that you feel sore and even have trouble sleeping at night. These are all symptoms of overtraining. In order to lose up to 10 pounds, you will need to do some form of exercise each day; however, you shouldn't aim for a high-intensity cardio or weight-lifting session every day. It's not realistic or good for your body, which needs periods of rest and recovery. Build one or two "light days" into your weekly workout schedule, but make them count! Schedule the same amount of time for your workout as a normal day, just exercise at a lower intensity. Light days might include biking, walking, dynamic stretching (walking lunges, trunk twists or arm circles, for instance), and swimming. Keep your body in motion but make sure you're giving hardworking muscles groups time to rest and recover so you're full of energy and stamina for your next tough workout.

Work toward your target heart rate

If you're not working out within your target heart rate zone, you're not getting the maximum benefits. The "fat burning zone," which burns the most calories and body fat stores, is reached at about 60 to 70 percent of your maximum heart rate. To calculate your maximum heart rate, subtract your age from 226 (for women, 220 for men). Then, multiply that number by 0.6 (60 percent) or 0.7 (70 percent) to find the number of beats per minute that is your target heart rate.

To determine whether you're in that zone during your workout, either wear a heart rate monitor or take your pulse

In addition to reps with weights, consider power yoga, which can burn more than 400 calories per hour and works multiple muscle groups at once. Yoga is a great workout because you're lifting your own body weight in many poses.

for 10 seconds and multiply the number of beats by 6. Adjust your intensity depending on whether you are above or below your target heart rate.

Exercise muscles in proper progression to maximize results.

When you're working a variety of muscles during a strength-training sequence, order is important. If your workout includes a variety of weightlifting exercises, begin with your larger muscle groups and move to the smaller muscles. This allows for optimal performance of the most demanding exercises when your fatigue levels are at their lowest and you feel energized and fresh. The most important thing is to be sure that you have enough energy to complete your entire workout. It is better to do less and complete the entire circuit than to neglect a muscle group or do an uneven number of reps from one side of the body to the other.

As your level of fitness improves, you should up the intensity of your workouts. For example, when running, aim for a sprinting pace of at least 7.5 mph, a running pace of at least 6.0 mph, and a jogging pace of at least 5.0 mph.

Variety is the spice of life

Variety helps keep you happy and motivated in both your diet and your workouts. If you restrict your diet to the point that you're eating only fish and salad, for instance, you'll quickly lose interest and enthusiasm.

Variety also keeps your weight loss and calorie burning from plateauing. If you do the same exercises, at the same intensity, day after day, working out will get boring and your body will stop burning fat and calories as quickly. You'll find your weight loss comes to a standstill. You need to plan for workouts that work different muscle groups at different intensities throughout the week. Because you're trying to torch through unwanted pounds, you'll want to focus on cardio but also complement it with strength training.

Carbs that are low in fat give you the energy you need to have a great workout. Protein helps with muscle repair and growth. Fat also acts as fuel for workouts, although you should eat mostly unsaturated fats.

In addition to reps with weights, consider power yoga, which can burn more than 400 calories per hour and works multiple muscle groups at once. Yoga is such a great workout because you're lifting your own body weight in many poses. Whatever you choose to do, creating a varied workout schedule is imperative to losing 10 pounds.

"Failure is not fatal, but failure to change might be.**"**

~ John Wooden

Chapter 13

Ultimate
Fitness Tips

You're well on your way to a successful diet and fitness program and, by now, you're seeing the weight drop off, feeling healthier, and enjoying more energy than ever. To continue making progress, you need to keep your body from plateauing and your dedication from waning.

To round out your program, you need a few powerful secrets. In this chapter, learn how to exercise efficiently, stay inspired, and breeze through physical activity on a daily basis, without your workout feeling like "work."

Motivation, seeing results, and enjoyment are the keys to sticking with a fitness plan for 2 weeks, or any amount of time. This book has given you all the tools you need to lose up to 10 pounds faster than you ever thought possible — use this final fitness chapter to rev up your workouts and get the very most from every minute of physical activity you do.

Make a music playlist to stay motivated

Music has been proven to help people work out longer and with more energy, as well as providing a distraction from fatigue. Dr. Costas Karageorghis, who has studied the effects of music on physical performance for 20 years, says that a good workout song should be between 120 and 140 beats-per-minute, which corresponds to the average person's heart rate while doing moderate exercise (up the tempo if you're working out harder). Most pop, rap, heavy metal and many rock songs fall into this tempo range. Even if it's not your favorite artist or a type of music that you'd listen to in your car, an upbeat song can help keep you going when your energy is low or you're nearing the end of a tough workout.

Work out with someone you see often, such as your neighbor, coworker, roommate or spouse, and you'll be best able to hold each other accountable.

Invest in new workout clothes

When you feel confident and have the proper exercise clothes, you will be more motivated to exercise, and you'll work out longer, too. Invest in a few new pieces of workout clothing and you'll be inspired and excited to wear them! Choose shirts, shorts, pants and sports bras in breathable, quick-drying fabrics that wick sweat away from the body. Exercise clothes should also stretch and move with you. Finally, be sure to get what you need for the specific activities you'll be doing, such as compression shorts for biking, form-fitting pants for yoga, and supportive undergarments for running.

Rehydrate and replenish with coconut water

Coconut water is one of the purest natural liquids around, second only to real water. It's one of nature's best superfoods! Unlike sugary sports drinks, coconut water contains natural electrolytes for energy and hydration but with minimal calories (typically about 60 per bottle). Coconut water has no added sugar and, with more potassium than a banana and 15 times more than most sports drinks, it prevents cramping and promotes muscle recovery during and after a workout. It also has myriad weight-loss benefits, such as increasing metabolism and promoting healthy thyroid function.

You can buy individual servings of coconut water at most health food stores and at many gyms and fitness studios. Its natural properties and benefits to your health and exercise program make it a favorite of cyclists, runners, trainers, yoginis, and more.

Use plyometrics to blast calories

Plyometrics are a great way to burn calories in a short amount of time. These types of exercise are designed to produce fast, powerful movements. The muscle is loaded and then contracted in rapid sequence. When these exercises are done in succession they burn calories quickly. Plyometrics are great because they are strength-building exercises that require endurance and cardiovascular stamina.

You can try mixing jump rope, jumping jacks, squat jumps, box jumps and other plyometric activities into your normal workouts, or refer to the *Lose Up to 10 Pounds in 2 Weeks Pocket Guide* exercise plan chapter in this book, which contains a complete, challenging plyometric workout.

Get Netflix

No one is recommending you sit on your couch with movies all night — but Netflix is actually a great, inexpensive way to work out at home! Their wide selection of exercise and fitness DVDs includes dance, aerobics, yoga, Pilates, strength training and more. Some DVDs are available for rental, delivered right to your mailbox and kept as long as you like, and others can be watched instantly online, or on a gaming console like Wii or Xbox. Workout DVDs are perfect for the times when you need a quick, 30-minute blast, don't have time to drive to the gym, or want to try something new in the privacy of your living room. Or, maybe you're not sure if Hollywood trainer Jillian Michaels' *30-Day Shred* is right for you? Netflix gives you the option to try specific exercise DVDs before buying them. Just be sure to type in the name of the video you want into the Search bar — the "Browse" feature shows only a very limited number of choices.

Did You Know?

According to a *Men's Fitness* magazine survey of more than 5,000 readers, guys' favorite part of a woman's body is her butt (40 percent), beating out legs and even breasts! Guys preferred voluptuous bodies, like Kim Kardashian's, and athletic bodies, like Cameron Diaz's, over stick-thin figures. All the more motivation to define curves and build sexy muscles.

Find a fitness buddy

Losing weight and getting active are always easier with a partner, so invite a spouse or friend to join you in your weight-loss efforts, especially if he or she seems threatened by or uncomfortable with your weight loss. The great things about a workout buddy is he or she keeps you accountable, motivated on the days when you don't feel like exercising, and keeps you company on hikes, bike rides, and rock climbing trips. Plus, if you're just trying out a new form of exercise, such as surfing or kickboxing, having a partner can make it more fun and less scary. Make your workout buddy someone you see often, such as your neighbor, coworker, roommate or spouse, and you'll be best able to hold each other accountable. You'll have

A good workout song should be between 120 and 140 beats-per-minute, which corresponds to the average person's heart rate while exercising.

someone to celebrate with when you both drop 10 pounds!

Schedule a cardio session around a TV show or sporting event

Running or bicycling for an hour or more in a gym can get dull fast. One tip for getting through a longer cardio session is to plan it for a time when a favorite show, movie or sporting event is on TV. Time will fly by when you're watching the Lakers game or an hour-long sitcom. Just be sure to do this when you have at least 45 minutes or more of cardio and you can work at a steady pace and zone out a bit. You won't want to be distracted by the TV screen if you're trying to get through 30 minutes of interval training, for instance.

Get a boost from pre-workout caffeine

The caffeine in natural sources such as coffee and green tea, or in pill form, benefits your workouts because it acts as a thermogenic. Themorgenics speed up your body's functions, including breath and heart rate, encouraging the body to use calories more quickly. Don't overdo it when it comes to caffeine, of course. Listen to your body, and if you feel lightheaded, dizzy or faint, stop what you're doing immediately, rest for a few minutes, and abstain from caffeine in the future. Otherwise, unless you're exercising at high altitudes or suffer from high blood pressure or another heart condition, taking 100 to 200 mg (one cup of coffee has about 100 mg) of caffeine 45 minutes before a workout can help you burn fat stores, speed up your metabolism, and help you power through a workout.

Count your steps with a pedometer

Start wearing a pedometer daily to measure how many steps you're taking and how many calories you're burning. Pedometers clip to your belt or pocket — or any spot where they will be perpendicular to the ground. They come in a variety of styles and price points — for less than $20 you can get a sleek, simple device that counts steps and calculates calories burned. Deluxe models play music, have audio features, and allow you to upload your daily stats into your computer to track your progress and meet goals. Many new mp3 players come with built-in pedometers, as well. You'll want to reference consumer reports that test the efficiency and accuracy of different makes and models.

For $99, a new Microsoft product called Fitbit accurately tracks your calories burned, steps taken, distance traveled and even sleep quality. On your Fitbit profile, you enter the calories you ate for the day and the data from your Fitbit device automatically calculates if you've met the distance and calorie goals you set for the day and week.

Drinking several cups of green tea can boost your workout and burns about 70 extra calories per day.

Blow off the gym!

Many people enjoy the routine schedule of going to the same location every day, but others find the gym stifling and somewhat limiting. Or, you may feel lost among the confusing machines, bustling trainers and intense gym rats. Be it burnout or pure intimidation, you may be looking for an alternative to the gym.

Naturally, getting outside in the fresh air is your best choice. If you live in a city where weather permits, add a fun activity to your weekly workout schedule — bike rides, hiking, surfing, horseback riding, rock climbing. Try something new to shake things up and stay motivated.

Caffeine benefits your workouts because it acts as a thermogenic. Themorgenics speed up your body's functions, including breath and heart rate, encouraging the body to use calories more quickly.

Bootcamps are also a great way to burn hundreds of calories in a short amount of time. Beach or park bootcamps are popping up all over the country, as well as indoor sessions that combine strength training with cardio. Bootcamps use interval training — bursts of activity with short rests in between exercises — to blast calories and fat. Another gym alternative is joining a private yoga or Pilates studio. You'll get focused, professional instructors and classes without the overwhelming nature of a gym atmosphere.

There are really hundreds of exercises, classes and groups available. Check out the website MeetUp.com to find out what's going on in your area. From surfing moms to salsa dancing clubs, if you can imagine it, it's out there.

> **"** It's not who you are that holds you back,
> it's who you think you're not. **"**
>
> ~ Unknown

Chapter 14

Activities & Calories Burned

All types of physical activity burn calories. You don't have to slave away at a gym — normal daily activities, chores and errands also require your body to burn calories, in addition to exercise.

This chapter highlights some of the typical physical activities, from sports to household chores, that you can do to burn calories while losing 10 pounds. They range from light to moderate to vigorous, so incorporate something from each list every day, or combine activities.

Be aware that the exact number of calories you will burn for each activity varies based on your weight. The following list is an approximation for someone who weighs 150 pounds. If you weigh more, you will burn slightly more calories; if you weigh less than 150 pounds, you will burn slightly fewer calories. If you require an exact count, there are many websites that can estimate calories burned based on your weight, intensity of the workout, and the length of time you exercised.

Light Activities: 150 or Less Cal/Hr.

Billiards 140
Lying down/sleeping 60
Office work 140
Sitting 80
Standing 100

Moderate Activities: 150-350 Cal/Hr.

Aerobic dancing 340
Ballroom dancing 210
Bicycling (5 mph) 170
Bowling 160
Canoeing (2.5 mph) 170
Dancing (social) 210
Gardening (moderate) 270
Golf (with cart) 180
Golf (without cart) 320
Grocery shopping 180
Horseback riding (sitting trot) 250
Light housework/cleaning, etc. 250
Pilates 240
Ping-pong 270
Surfing 300
Swimming (20 yards/min) 290
Tennis (recreational doubles) 310
Vacuuming 220
Volleyball (recreational) 260
Walking (2 mph) 200
Walking (3 mph) 240
Walking (4 mph) 300

Vigorous Activities: 350 or More Cal/Hr.

Aerobics (step) 440
Backpacking (10 lb load). 540
Badminton 450
Basketball (competitive) 660
Basketball (leisure) 390
Bicycling (10 mph) 375
Bicycling (13 mph) 600
Cross country skiing (leisurely). 460
Cross country skiing (moderate). 660
Hiking 460
Ice skating (9 mph) 384
Jogging (5 mph) 550
Jogging (6 mph) 690
Racquetball. 620
Rock Climbing 740
Rollerblading 384
Rowing machine. 540
Running (8 mph). 900
Scuba diving 570
Shoveling snow 580
Soccer 580
Spinning 650
Stair climber machine. 480
Swimming (50 yards/min.) 680
Water aerobics 400
Water skiing 480
Weight training (30 sec. between sets) 760
Weight training (60 sec. between sets) 570
Yoga (Power). 400

The greatest wealth is health.

~ Virgil

Chapter 15

Lose Up to
10 Pounds in 2 Weeks
Exercise Plan

Losing weight requires a fitness plan full of high-intensity, calorie-blasting exercises that work the whole body. The *Lose Up to 10 Pounds in 2 Weeks Pocket Guide* exercise plan is designed to target multiple muscle groups, build core strength, and get the heart rate elevated to burn body fat.

Six days out of each week you will pair a strength training circuit with a cardio circuit. You won't need any props or weights — just water to drink, stable exercise shoes, and moveable, breathable workout clothing. You will switch off each day between an upper body and core strength training circuit and a lower body and core strength training circuit. You will also alternate between a plyometric cardio circuit and a kickboxing cardio circuit. The last day of the week is to rest.

Every strength training exercise comes with step-by-step instructions, as well as modifications to make the move easier or harder. You may want to challenge yourself more on some exercises, or modify some moves to avoid injury or account for soreness.

For the cardio circuits, you will be able to work faster and harder without sacrificing form as your fitness level improves.

How to Do the Exercise Plan

You will need to set aside about 60 minutes to complete this workout plan. Do each exercise for 50 seconds, as many reps as you can do in that time without sacrificing form. Take a 10-second rest to get ready for the next exercise. Keep your eye on a stopwatch, timer on an mp3 player, or clock with a seconds hand. Complete all 6 exercises in the strength training circuit, then repeat the full circuit for a second round, and again for a third round. After you have completed 3 rounds of the strength training circuit, take a 2-minute water break and move on to the cardio circuit. Do the same for the cardio circuit.

Warming Up and Cooling Down

Always begin and end your strength training and cardio workouts with a 5- to 10-minute warm-up and cool-down. Walk, lightly jog or run in place to loosen the muscles. Next, stretch to prepare your muscles for work and prevent injury.

Important stretches include holding the heel close to the glute to stretch the quad muscle, reaching toward the toes to stretch hamstrings, calf stretches against a wall, and stretching your arms behind your head and across the chest to loosen shoulders, chest, biceps and triceps.

The same routine after your workout will bring the heart rate down, help the body recover and prevent soreness.

Your Workout Schedule

You only have 2 short weeks to get the body you've always wanted, so work hard and push yourself, even if it's to do one more rep! You'll love the feeling of success and pride you'll get after a tough workout. The body, strength and shape you've always wanted is just a couple of weeks away.

WEEK 1	STRENGTH	CARDIO
Mon	Upper Body & Core	Plyometrics
Tues	Lower Body & Core	Kickboxing
Wed	Upper Body & Core	Plyometrics
Thurs	Lower Body & Core	Kickboxing
Fri	Upper Body & Core	Plyometrics
Sat	Lower Body & Core	Kickboxing
Sun	Rest Day!	Rest Day!

WEEK 2	STRENGTH	CARDIO
Mon	Upper Body & Core	Kickboxing
Tues	Lower Body & Core	Plyometrics
Wed	Upper Body & Core	Kickboxing
Thurs	Lower Body & Core	Plyometrics
Fri	Upper Body & Core	Kickboxing
Sat	Lower Body & Core	Plyometrics
Sun	Rest Day!	Rest Day!

Notes:

UPPER BODY & CORE

CHEST, ARMS, SHOULDERS, BACK & CORE

Strength training is a very important part of losing weight. It lengthens and tones your body while replacing body fat with muscle, which burns three times as many calories as fat.

The exercises in this section work the upper body, including the chest, arms, shoulders, back and core. When coupled with the cardio programs described later in this chapter, you will get in shape quickly. Plus, they're fun and challenging!

JUDO PUSHUPS

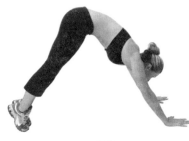

1 Put your hands and feet on the ground with hips lifted so your body forms an inverted V shape.

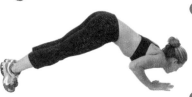

2 Keeping your hips up, bend your arms out to the side, and lower your upper body until your chin is near the floor.

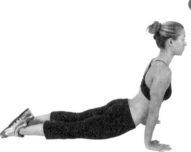

3 Lower your hips toward the floor while you lift your upper body simultaneously. Then slide back into the original position, reversing the way you went in, for one rep.

Make It Easier: Put your knees on the ground as you lower your hips to the floor.

Make It Harder: Lift one leg.

BURPEES

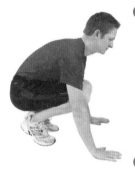

❶ Begin standing. Drop into a squat position with hands on the floor in front of you.

❷ Kick your feet back into a pushup position without letting your hips sag.

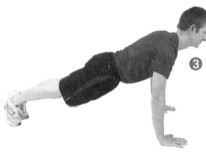

❸ Immediately jump your feet back to the squat position; then jump straight up as high as you can for one complete rep.

Make It Easier: Walk your feet back into pushup position.

Make It Harder: Move as quickly as you can through the reps. Jump as high as you can each time.

SIDE PLANK W/ PUSHUP

1 Start in plank position.

2 Flip to one side; straighten your bottom arm directly under your shoulder, legs straight, and feet stacked. Place your free hand on your hip or stretch it up. Keep your back straight and do not allow your hips to sag. Work on tightening your abs and lifting your side away from the ground.

3 Flip back to plank and complete a pushup.

Make It Easier: Place one knee on the ground when you flip to the side.

Make It Harder: Lift the top leg up in side plank.

ARMS DIPS

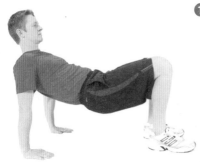

1 Position your hands shoulder-width apart on the floor behind you and place feet hip-width apart on the floor in front of you.

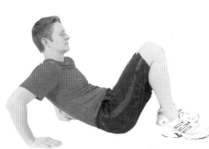

2 Lift your hips so you are in a crab-like position. Bend your elbows and lower your hips down toward the floor. Then, press into your hands back up to your starting position. Don't straighten your arms all the way; keep your elbows slightly bent to keep tension on the arm muscles.

Make It Easier: Move your feet closer to your body.

Make It Harder: Straighten your legs out in front of you.

BENT KNEE V-UP

1 Lie on the floor with arms straight alongside the body and legs out straight.

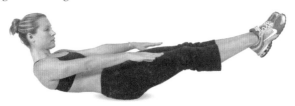

2 Simultaneously, lift your chest and bring your knees toward the chest in a crunch. Lower back toward the starting position for one rep.

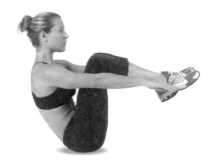

Make It Easier: Keep the back and shoulders on the ground and bring knees up into the body.

Make It Harder: Do a V Up by simultaneously lifting your arms and legs straight up in a V shape as if trying to touch your toes at the top.

REACHING PLANK

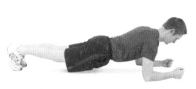

1 Position yourself face down and prop yourself up on your elbows, forearms, and toes in a plank position. Maintain a flat back and tighten your abs so the hips don't sag.

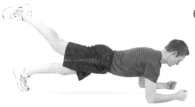

2 Next, inhale and lift one leg, lengthening and holding for a few seconds.

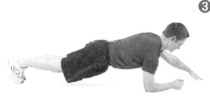

3 Return to plank, and reach out in front of your body with your opposite hand. Switch and perform on the other leg.

Make It Easier: Skip the reach. Or, bend knees and place them on the ground.

Make It Harder: Lift the leg higher and squeeze the glutes. Don't let your hips sag.

Notes:

LOWER BODY

LEGS, GLUTES & CORE

These lower body exercises will whip your legs, glutes and core into shape in just 2 weeks. You'll feel leaner, stronger and more explosive, especially when you combine these moves with the cardio exercises described later in this chapter.

Don't forget to challenge yourself as much as possible, and modify as necessary to push yourself or account for injuries or sore muscles.

WIDE SQUATS

❶ Stand with feet wide, toes turned out slightly, with hands together at chest height.

❷ Squat low to the ground, squeezing the glutes. As you come up, lift your arms over your head until they are straight, for one complete rep. Be sure to keep the core engaged and don't hunch forward. Push through the feet to rise up and return to starting position.

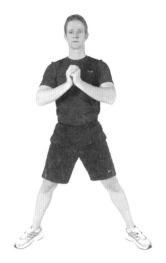

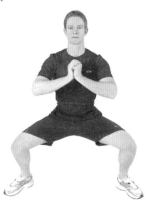

Make It Easier: Don't sink as low to the ground.

Make It Harder: Go slowly, and focus the weight into your heels.

LUNGES WITH A TWIST

1 Start standing, then step forward into a lunge, making sure your knee doesn't go past your toes.

2 When you reach the lowest point of your lunge, twist your torso to the side, squeezing the core. Stand up from the lunge and repeat on the other leg. Keep your back straight and your thigh parallel to the ground in your lunge.

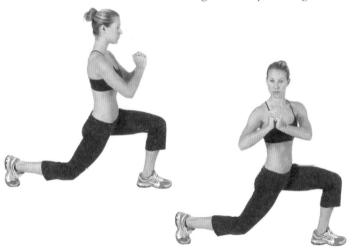

Make It Easier: Don't sink as low in your lunge.

Make It Harder: Twist and lunge slowly and more deeply.

BRIDGE POSE

1 Lie flat with knees bent and hip-width apart; tuck your pelvis so your lower back touches the floor.

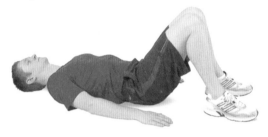

2 Raise your hips until your body forms a straight line from shoulders to knees. Squeeze your glutes, engage abs, and elevate through the thighs. Hold for 2 to 5 seconds and lower to the floor.

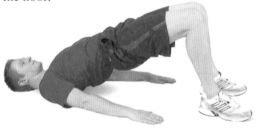

Make It Easier: Move your feet away from your body.

Make It Harder: Pull your feet as close to your body as you can. Lift one leg and hold for a few seconds. Lower and lift the other leg before returning to start position.

BICYCLES

1 Lie on your back with your knees bent at a 90-degree angle.

2 Lace your fingers behind your head. Lift your head and shoulders, exhale and twist to one side, bringing your knee in toward your opposite elbow, while straightening the other leg. Return to center, inhale.

3 Exhale and twist to the opposite side.

Make It Easier: Keep feet on the ground and slide heels along the floor using a towel.

Make It Harder: Perform bicycles as fast as you can, being sure to rotate from the core.

FIRE HYDRANT

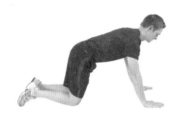

1 Get on the floor on your hands and knees with a flat back, in a table position.

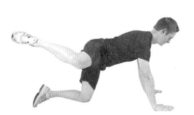

2 Keeping your knee bent, lift one knee up and out to the side. Try to lift the knee as high as your hip, or whatever height is comfortable, squeezing the glutes.

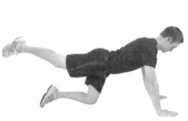

3 Next, kick the raised leg back until it is straight behind you. Lower the leg to the starting position and repeat, switching legs at the 25-second mark.

Make It Easier: Skip the kick back.

Make It Harder: Raise the leg higher, squeezing the glutes.

RUSSIAN TWIST

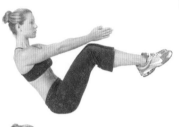

① Sit with your legs bent. Hold arms out in front of you and press the palms together. Lean slightly back so your upper body forms a 45-degree angle with the floor and lift your feet off the floor.

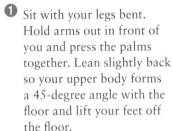

② Rotate your arms with palms pressed as far to one side as you can, reaching over while you squeeze your abs and obliques.

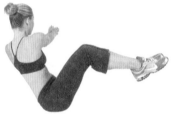

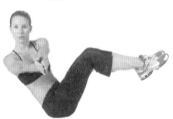

③ Return to center and twist to the other side. Keep your feet lifted and centered; rotate from your core, not your hips.

Make It Easier: Keep your feet flat on the ground.

Make It Harder: Cycle your legs as you twist. When you twist to the right, extend your left leg and pull your right knee into your chest; repeat on the other side. Don't let your feet touch the floor at any point.

Notes:

_____

_____

_____

_____

_____

_____

_____

_____

_____

_____

_____

_____

_____

_____

_____

_____

_____

_____

_____

_____

PLYOMETRICS

Plyometrics are a great way to build muscle, burn a lot of calories in a short amount of time, and get your heart rate up.

During all plyometric exercises it is important to keep knees slightly bent when pushing off and landing. Never land with a thud; think of exploding out, using your muscles to coil and spring. Be sure to stretch well and warm up and cool down before and after this circuit.

JUMPING JACKS

1 Stand with feet together and arms by your sides.

2 Jump legs out to the sides, simultaneously raising arms overhead; then immediately jump back to the starting position. Repeat as fast as you can, focusing on controlling the arms and legs.

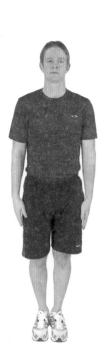
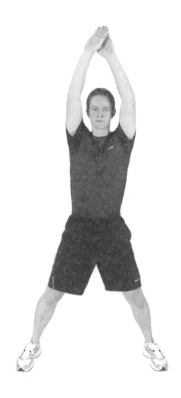

SPLIT JUMPS

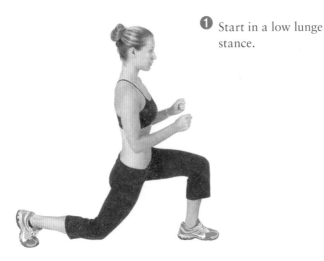

❶ Start in a low lunge stance.

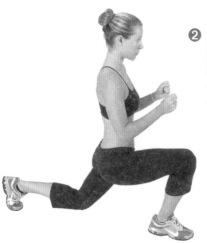

❷ Bend the knees and jump, switching legs to land in the same position on the opposite leg. Go as quickly as you can without sacrificing form.

HIGH KNEES

❶ Bend your arms at 90-degree angles and hold them out in front of you, palms down.

❷ Start running in place, lifting the knees as high as your palms. Running on the toes will make this exercise more beneficial. Make sure you don't lean too far back. Repeat as fast as you can.

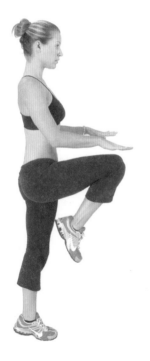
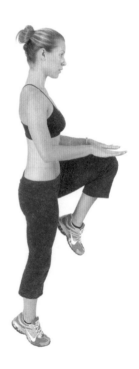

STAR JUMP

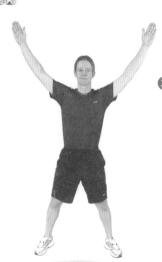

1 Stand with your knees slightly bent.

2 Squat down and get ready to explode out.

3 Jump as high as you can, stretching your arms and legs out to the sides in a star shape in the air. Before you land, pull your arms and legs back to your body, landing in the starting position. Repeat with little to no rest between jumps.

LATERAL JUMP

❶ Choose a low, flat object you can jump over, such as a broomstick or jump rope. Start standing on one side.

❷ Jump sideways to opposite side of the object, then immediately jump back to other side and repeat as quickly as possible.

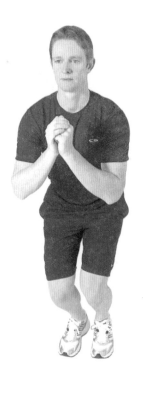
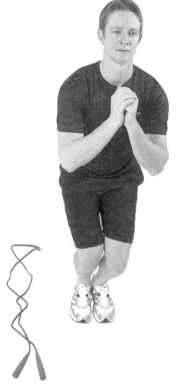

MOUNTAIN CLIMBERS

1 Begin in a pushup position with arms straight. Bring one knee in toward the chest, placing the toe on the floor.

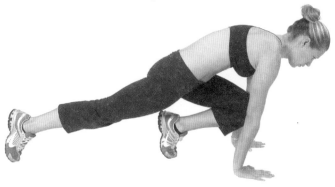

2 Jump and switch legs in the air, bringing the back foot in and the front foot back. Continue alternating the feet as fast as you can without sacrificing form.

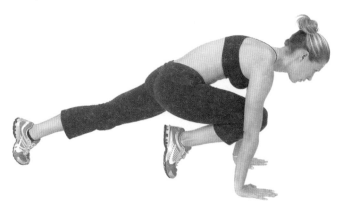

Notes:

_____

_____

_____

_____

_____

_____

_____

_____

_____

_____

_____

_____

_____

_____

_____

_____

_____

_____

_____

_____

_____

_____

KICKBOXING

This fast fat-burning workout is fun and dynamic, and it improves cardio conditioning and increases endurance. It can be done anywhere, just be sure you have ample room for kicks and jabs at full extension. Keep abs engaged throughout the entire sequence and don't sacrifice form for speed. Inhale before you kick or jab and exhale during the kick or jab.

Be sure to walk for a few minutes or jog in place to warm up the body for this cardio plan.

FRONT KICK

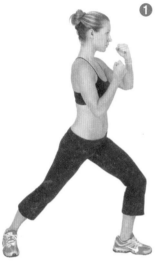

❶ Stand with left foot forward in fighting stance, fists up. Begin to shift your weight to the left foot.

❷ Kick straight out as if you were reaching with the ball of the foot. Retract immediately and return to fighting stance. Do as many kicks with the right leg as you can and switch to the left leg halfway through at the 25-second mark.

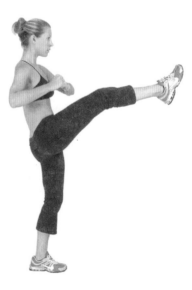

UPPERCUT

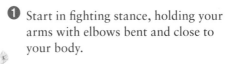

❶ Start in fighting stance, holding your arms with elbows bent and close to your body.

❷ Get low for power, and step into the punch, pushing your left fist up. Remember to push through your legs.

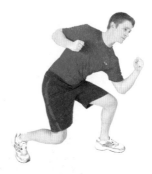

❸ Recoil and repeat, switching arms halfway through, at the 25-second mark.

KNEE KICK

1 Begin in fighting stance, with the kicking leg back. Reach up with your arms, as if pulling an imaginary opponent toward you, and drive your knee up, keeping your toes pointed down. Bend your bottom leg slightly for leverage.

2 Drop the kicking leg back down, and repeat, alternating legs halfway through at the 25-second mark.

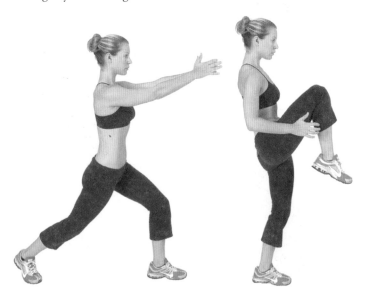

SIDE KICK

1 Start in a horse stance, with feet slightly wider than shoulder-width apart, feet pointing forward, and knees slightly bent and out to the side.

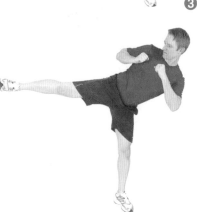

2 Lift your right knee toward your chest, keeping your foot flexed.

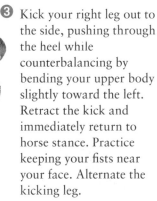

3 Kick your right leg out to the side, pushing through the heel while counterbalancing by bending your upper body slightly toward the left. Retract the kick and immediately return to horse stance. Practice keeping your fists near your face. Alternate the kicking leg.

RIGHT & LEFT PUNCH

1 Stand with left foot forward in fighting stance, with fists up.

2 Pivot your right hip forward, extending and jabbing with the right arm. Your fist should be parallel to the floor at full extension, and your arm should be in line with your shoulder.

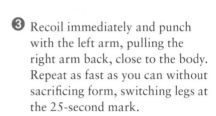

3 Recoil immediately and punch with the left arm, pulling the right arm back, close to the body. Repeat as fast as you can without sacrificing form, switching legs at the 25-second mark.

BACK KICK

1 Stand in fighting stance.

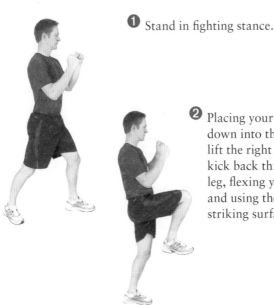

2 Placing your weight down into the front leg, lift the right knee, then kick back through that leg, flexing your foot and using the heel as a striking surface.

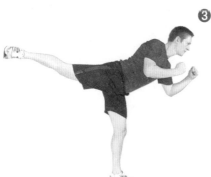

3 Lower your leg back to the starting position. Do as many kicks with the right leg as you can and switch to the left leg halfway through at the 25-second mark.

The secret of health for both mind and body is not to mourn for the past, nor to worry about the future, but to live the present moment wisely and earnestly.

~ Buddha

Chapter 16

How to Use the Journal Pages

These journal pages are an instrumental part of losing 10 pounds in 2 weeks because they help you monitor your weight, calorie intake, and calories burned through exercise. The best way to create a significant calorie deficit per day is to plan ahead and create a calorie "budget" for each meal and snack and determine how much exercise you need to burn additional calories. Anticipating how many calories you can "spend" at each meal takes the guesswork out of cooking and ordering off restaurant menus. For instance, if you have 400 calories to budget for lunch, you may decide to order a turkey sub with cheese and spend the whole amount, or you may opt for the veggie sub with no cheese and save 150 calories.

The journal pages also give you clues into how food, exercise and hydration factor into your mood and energy levels. You may find fascinating correlations between what and when you're eating and how great or lousy you're feeling. Plus, nothing is a better motivator for exercise than realizing how much more energy and stamina you have throughout the day when you've hit the gym or gone for a bike ride.

Another great benefit of a diet and fitness journal is it keeps you accountable. It's easy to let a 150-calorie cookie slip your mind, or to tell yourself you worked out for 30 minutes when it was really only 20, but those little white lies are much more difficult when you're recording everything in a journal throughout the day. You've likely put on extra weight by not holding yourself accountable in the past; this journal will help you break that bad habit and start keeping track of everything you eat, drink and do by way of exercise. It's the proven way to slim down faster!

Here is an explanation of the different components of the journal pages:

❶ **DAILY NUTRITIONAL INTAKE:** Record your daily intake of calories, fats and carbs for each meal and snack. Write down your totals for breakfast, lunch, dinner, and two snacks. Compare these totals to your nutritional intake goal from earlier in this book and see if you are meeting or going over your target amounts. There is also a column called "Other" that can be used to track intake of protein, fiber, sugar, sodium or another nutrient if you have special dietary concerns, such as high blood pressure or diabetes.

❷ **WATER INTAKE:** Strive for at least eight 8-ounce glasses of water per day. Check off a box for each glass you drink. If you drink water on a regular basis throughout the day, your metabolism works faster and better and you'll have more energy for exercise.

❸ **DAILY NUMBER OF SERVINGS:** At the end of each day, write down the number of servings you ate from each of the six major food groups. Eating a balanced diet is a big part of losing weight and keeping it off.

❹ **VITAMINS & SUPPLEMENTS:** Make note of the vitamins or supplements you are including in your program. When in doubt about specific vitamin recommendations, consult with a health care professional.

⑤ DAILY GOAL: Write down a goal each day and try your best to stick to it. When you do meet your daily goal, check off the box and you can feel proud of your success!

⑥ PHYSICAL ACTIVITY: Record all physical activity you do, including cardio, strength training, flexibility training, or a combination of all three. Record the duration, distance, pace, weight, sets, number of repetitions, and total calories burned.

⑦ CALORIE CALCULATOR: This formula helps you find your Daily Net Calorie Gain or Loss for each day. Start with your Total Calorie Intake for that day, subtract the Total Calories Burned from physical activity to get Net Calories. Then, subtract your BMR (the number of calories your body burns at rest, calculated earlier in this book) to get your Daily Net Calorie Gain or Loss. Your goal is for this to be a negative number, meaning you created a calorie deficit, which is necessary to lose weight.

⑧ ENERGY LEVEL: Document your daily overall energy by rating your energy levels from 1 to 6. Take note of how your energy correlates to the types of foods you have eaten that day. For example, if you notice that a little extra protein helps you get through your workout with more energy, incorporate lean meats in your diet. As you discover these relationships, make adjustments as needed to help you feel your best.

⑨ MUSCLE GROUP WORKED: Document which of the 6 major muscle groups you work each day during exercise. Strive to include workouts that work your entire body, but also pay attention to how your body feels and give certain muscle groups sufficient rest to prevent injury.

Sample Journal Page

DIET JOURNAL

Day 1 ❶ DATE: _Feb. 2_   WEIGHT: _197_

BREAKFAST	Qty.	Calories	Fat	Carbs	Protein/Other
Blueberry scone	1	400	17	55	5
Orange juice	12oz.	110	0	26	2

SNACK	Qty.	Calories	Fat	Carbs	Other
Baby carrots		100	0	24	3

LUNCH	Qty.	Calories	Fat	Carbs	Other
Bagel w/turkey		490	4	70	30
American cheese	2	64	2	2	8
Pepsi	12oz.	180	0	45	0

SNACK	Qty.	Calories	Fat	Carbs	Other
PB + apple slices		245	17	21	10

DINNER	Qty.	Calories	Fat	Carbs	Other
Salmon	8oz.	416	22	0	45
Wild rice		166	2	34	7
Broccoli		54	1	12	2
Crystal Light tea		5	0	0	0

DAILY INTAKE TOTALS:	2,230	65	289	112

✓ Water Intake ❷
# of 8 oz. glasses

☑ ☑ ☑
☑ ☑ ☑
☑ ☑ ☐

Daily # of Servings ❸

3 fruits
2 veggies
3 grains

2 meats & beans
1 milk & dairy
3 oils & sweets

Vitamins & Supplements: ❹

Calcium
Vitamin C

FITNESS JOURNAL

❺ DAILY GOAL: _Eat a high-protein dinner_ ————— **GOAL MET:** ☑

❻ 🏃 CARDIOVASCULAR EXERCISE	Duration	Distance	Pace	Cal. Burned
Shooting the basketball	60 mins		medium	300
Jogging	20 mins	1.5 mi	4.5mph	205

🏋 STRENGTH TRAINING	Weight	Reps.	Sets	Cal. Burned
Bicep curls	25	3	36	20
Pull-ups		2	8	25
Push-ups		2	60	35

🧘 FLEXIBILITY, RELAXATION, MEDITATION	Duration	Cal. Burned
Stretching	10 mins	5

❼ DAILY CALORIES BURNED: 590

CALORIE CALCULATOR

2,230	−	590	=	1,640	−	1,979	=	−339
TOTAL CALORIE INTAKE		TOTAL CALORIES BURNED		NET CALORIES		BMR (Basal Metabolic Rate)		DAILY NET CALORIE GAIN OR LOSS

❽ Energy Level:
👎 1 2 3 4 ⑤ 6 👍

❾ Muscle Group Worked:
☑ arms ☑ chest ☐ back ☐ core ☑ thighs ☑ calves

Diet & Workout Notes:

Need more fiber during breakfast! Buy oatmeal. Do 45 minutes of cardio tomorrow.

Day 1   DATE: _____   WEIGHT: _____

⭕ BREAKFAST	Qty.	Calories	Fat	Carbs	Other
_____	___				
_____	___				
_____	___				
_____	___				

➕ SNACK	Qty.	Calories	Fat	Carbs	Other
_____	___				

🥪 LUNCH	Qty.	Calories	Fat	Carbs	Other
_____	___				
_____	___				
_____	___				
_____	___				

🍇 SNACK	Qty.	Calories	Fat	Carbs	Other
_____	___				

🥄 DINNER	Qty.	Calories	Fat	Carbs	Other
_____	___				
_____	___				
_____	___				
_____	___				

DAILY INTAKE TOTALS:

✓ **Water Intake**
# of 8 oz. glasses

☐ ☐ ☐
☐ ☐ ☐
☐ ☐ ☐

Daily # of Servings

☐ fruits   ☐ meats & beans

☐ veggies   ☐ milk & dairy

☐ grains   ☐ oils & sweets

Vitamins & Supplements:

_____

_____

_____

FITNESS JOURNAL

DAILY GOAL: _____ GOAL MET: ☐

🏃 CARDIOVASCULAR EXERCISE

	Duration	Distance	Pace	Cal. Burned
_____				
_____				
_____				

🏋 STRENGTH TRAINING

	Weight	Reps.	Sets	Cal. Burned
_____				
_____				
_____				
_____				
_____				
_____				

🧘 FLEXIBILITY, RELAXATION, MEDITATION

	Duration	Cal. Burned
_____		
_____		

DAILY CALORIES BURNED: _____

CALORIE CALCULATOR

TOTAL CALORIE INTAKE	−	TOTAL CALORIES BURNED	=	NET CALORIES	−	BMR (Basal Metabolic Rate)	=	DAILY NET CALORIE GAIN OR LOSS

Energy Level:
👎 1 2 3 4 5 6 👍

Muscle Group Worked:
☐ arms ☐ chest ☐ back ☐ core ☐ thighs ☐ calves

Diet & Workout Notes:

_____

_____

DIET JOURNAL

Day 2   DATE: _____   WEIGHT: _____

BREAKFAST	Qty.	Calories	Fat	Carbs	Other

SNACK	Qty.	Calories	Fat	Carbs	Other

LUNCH	Qty.	Calories	Fat	Carbs	Other

SNACK	Qty.	Calories	Fat	Carbs	Other

DINNER	Qty.	Calories	Fat	Carbs	Other

DAILY INTAKE TOTALS:

✓ **Water Intake**
# of 8 oz. glasses

Daily # of Servings

	fruits		meats & beans
	veggies		milk & dairy
	grains		oils & sweets

Vitamins & Supplements:
_____
_____
_____

FITNESS JOURNAL

DAILY GOAL: _____ GOAL MET: ☐

CARDIOVASCULAR EXERCISE

	Duration	Distance	Pace	Cal. Burned

STRENGTH TRAINING

	Weight	Reps.	Sets	Cal. Burned

FLEXIBILITY, RELAXATION, MEDITATION

	Duration	Cal. Burned

DAILY CALORIES BURNED:

CALORIE CALCULATOR

TOTAL CALORIE INTAKE	−	TOTAL CALORIES BURNED	=	NET CALORIES	−	BMR (Basal Metabolic Rate)	=	DAILY NET CALORIE GAIN OR LOSS

Energy Level: 1 2 3 4 5 6

Muscle Group Worked: ☐ arms ☐ chest ☐ back ☐ core ☐ thighs ☐ calves

Diet & Workout Notes:

_____

_____

DIET JOURNAL

Day 3   DATE: _____   WEIGHT: _____

🍎 BREAKFAST

	Qty.	Calories	Fat	Carbs	Other
_____	___				
_____	___				
_____	___				
_____	___				

⊕ SNACK

	Qty.	Calories	Fat	Carbs	Other
_____	___				

🍞 LUNCH

	Qty.	Calories	Fat	Carbs	Other
_____	___				
_____	___				
_____	___				
_____	___				

🍪 SNACK

	Qty.	Calories	Fat	Carbs	Other
_____	___				

🍳 DINNER

	Qty.	Calories	Fat	Carbs	Other
_____	___				
_____	___				
_____	___				
_____	___				

DAILY INTAKE TOTALS:

✓ **Water Intake**
# of 8 oz. glasses

☐ ☐ ☐
☐ ☐ ☐

Daily # of Servings

	fruits		meats & beans
	veggies		milk & dairy
	grains		oils & sweets

Vitamins & Supplements:

_____
_____
_____

FITNESS JOURNAL

DAILY GOAL: _____ GOAL MET: ☐

🏃 CARDIOVASCULAR EXERCISE

	Duration	Distance	Pace	Cal. Burned

🏋 STRENGTH TRAINING

	Weight	Reps.	Sets	Cal. Burned

🧘 FLEXIBILITY, RELAXATION, MEDITATION

	Duration	Cal. Burned

DAILY CALORIES BURNED: _____

CALORIE CALCULATOR

	−		=		−		=	
TOTAL CALORIE INTAKE		TOTAL CALORIES BURNED		NET CALORIES		BMR (Basal Metabolic Rate)		DAILY NET CALORIE GAIN OR LOSS

Energy Level:
👎 1 2 3 4 5 6 👍

Muscle Group Worked: ☐ arms ☐ chest ☐ back ☐ core ☐ thighs ☐ calves

Diet & Workout Notes:

_____

_____

DIET JOURNAL

Day 4   DATE: _____   WEIGHT: _____

BREAKFAST	Qty.	Calories	Fat	Carbs	Other

SNACK	Qty.	Calories	Fat	Carbs	Other

LUNCH	Qty.	Calories	Fat	Carbs	Other

SNACK	Qty.	Calories	Fat	Carbs	Other

DINNER	Qty.	Calories	Fat	Carbs	Other

DAILY INTAKE TOTALS:

✓ **Water Intake**
# of 8 oz. glasses

Daily # of Servings

fruits   meats & beans

veggies   milk & dairy

grains   oils & sweets

Vitamins & Supplements:
_____
_____
_____

FITNESS JOURNAL

DAILY GOAL:_____ GOAL MET: ☐

🏃 CARDIOVASCULAR EXERCISE

	Duration	Distance	Pace	Cal. Burned

🏋 STRENGTH TRAINING

	Weight	Reps.	Sets	Cal. Burned

🧘 FLEXIBILITY, RELAXATION, MEDITATION

	Duration	Cal. Burned

DAILY CALORIES BURNED:

CALORIE CALCULATOR

	−		=		−		=	
TOTAL CALORIE INTAKE		TOTAL CALORIES BURNED		NET CALORIES		BMR (Basal Metabolic Rate)		DAILY NET CALORIE GAIN OR LOSS

Energy Level: 👎 1 2 3 4 5 6 👍

Muscle Group Worked: ☐ arms ☐ chest ☐ back ☐ core ☐ thighs ☐ calves

Diet & Workout Notes:

_____

_____

Day 5   DATE: _____   WEIGHT: _____

BREAKFAST	Qty.	Calories	Fat	Carbs	Other
_____	___				
_____	___				
_____	___				
_____	___				

SNACK	Qty.	Calories	Fat	Carbs	Other
_____	___				

LUNCH	Qty.	Calories	Fat	Carbs	Other
_____	___				
_____	___				
_____	___				
_____	___				

SNACK	Qty.	Calories	Fat	Carbs	Other
_____	___				

DINNER	Qty.	Calories	Fat	Carbs	Other
_____	___				
_____	___				
_____	___				
_____	___				

DAILY INTAKE TOTALS:

✓ **Water Intake**
# of 8 oz. glasses

☐ ☐ ☐
☐ ☐ ☐
☐ ☐ ☐

Daily # of Servings

fruits

veggies

grains

meats & beans

milk & dairy

oils & sweets

Vitamins & Supplements:

_____

_____

_____

FITNESS JOURNAL

DAILY GOAL: _____ GOAL MET: ☐

CARDIOVASCULAR EXERCISE	Duration	Distance	Pace	Cal. Burned
_____				
_____				
_____•_____				

STRENGTH TRAINING	Weight	Reps.	Sets	Cal. Burned
_____				
_____				
_____				
_____				
_____				
_____				
_____				

FLEXIBILITY, RELAXATION, MEDITATION	Duration	Cal. Burned
_____		
_____		

DAILY CALORIES BURNED: _____

CALORIE CALCULATOR

	–		=		–		=	
TOTAL CALORIE INTAKE		TOTAL CALORIES BURNED		NET CALORIES		BMR (Basal Metabolic Rate)		DAILY NET CALORIE GAIN OR LOSS

Energy Level: 👎 1 2 3 4 5 6 👍

Muscle Group Worked: ☐ arms ☐ chest ☐ back ☐ core ☐ thighs ☐ calves

Diet & Workout Notes:

_____

_____

Day 6   DATE: _____   WEIGHT: _____

BREAKFAST	Qty.	Calories	Fat	Carbs	Other

SNACK	Qty.	Calories	Fat	Carbs	Other

LUNCH	Qty.	Calories	Fat	Carbs	Other

SNACK	Qty.	Calories	Fat	Carbs	Other

DINNER	Qty.	Calories	Fat	Carbs	Other

DAILY INTAKE TOTALS:

✓ **Water Intake**
# of 8 oz. glasses

Daily # of Servings

fruits   meats & beans

veggies   milk & dairy

grains   oils & sweets

Vitamins & Supplements:

FITNESS JOURNAL

DAILY GOAL:_____ GOAL MET: ☐

CARDIOVASCULAR EXERCISE

	Duration	Distance	Pace	Cal. Burned

STRENGTH TRAINING

	Weight	Reps.	Sets	Cal. Burned

FLEXIBILITY, RELAXATION, MEDITATION

	Duration	Cal. Burned

DAILY CALORIES BURNED:

CALORIE CALCULATOR

	−		=		−		=	
TOTAL CALORIE INTAKE		TOTAL CALORIES BURNED		NET CALORIES		BMR (Basal Metabolic Rate)		DAILY NET CALORIE GAIN OR LOSS

Energy Level: 1 2 3 4 5 6

Muscle Group Worked: ☐ arms ☐ chest ☐ back ☐ core ☐ thighs ☐ calves

Diet & Workout Notes:

_____

_____

Day 7

DATE: _____   WEIGHT:_____

BREAKFAST	Qty.	Calories	Fat	Carbs	Other

SNACK	Qty.	Calories	Fat	Carbs	Other

LUNCH	Qty.	Calories	Fat	Carbs	Other

SNACK	Qty.	Calories	Fat	Carbs	Other

DINNER	Qty.	Calories	Fat	Carbs	Other

DAILY INTAKE TOTALS:

✓ **Water Intake**
# of 8 oz. glasses

☐ ☐ ☐
☐ ☐ ☐
☐ ☐ ☐

Daily # of Servings

fruits

veggies

grains

meats & beans

milk & dairy

oils & sweets

Vitamins & Supplements:

_____

_____

_____

FITNESS JOURNAL

DAILY GOAL: _____ GOAL MET: ☐

🏃 CARDIOVASCULAR EXERCISE

	Duration	Distance	Pace	Cal. Burned

🏋 STRENGTH TRAINING

	Weight	Reps.	Sets	Cal. Burned

🧘 FLEXIBILITY, RELAXATION, MEDITATION

	Duration	Cal. Burned

DAILY CALORIES BURNED:

CALORIE CALCULATOR

TOTAL CALORIE INTAKE	−	TOTAL CALORIES BURNED	=	NET CALORIES	−	BMR (Basal Metabolic Rate)	=	DAILY NET CALORIE GAIN OR LOSS

Energy Level: 👎 1 2 3 4 5 6 👍

Muscle Group Worked: ☐ arms ☐ chest ☐ back ☐ core ☐ thighs ☐ calves

Diet & Workout Notes:

_____

_____

DIET JOURNAL

Day 8   DATE: _____   WEIGHT: _____

BREAKFAST	Qty.	Calories	Fat	Carbs	Other

SNACK	Qty.	Calories	Fat	Carbs	Other

LUNCH	Qty.	Calories	Fat	Carbs	Other

SNACK	Qty.	Calories	Fat	Carbs	Other

DINNER	Qty.	Calories	Fat	Carbs	Other

DAILY INTAKE TOTALS:

✓ **Water Intake**
# of 8 oz. glasses

Daily # of Servings

fruits   meats & beans

veggies   milk & dairy

grains   oils & sweets

Vitamins & Supplements:

_____

_____

_____

FITNESS JOURNAL

DAILY GOAL: _____ GOAL MET: ☐

CARDIOVASCULAR EXERCISE

	Duration	Distance	Pace	Cal. Burned
_____				
_____				
_____				

STRENGTH TRAINING

	Weight	Reps.	Sets	Cal. Burned
_____				
_____				
_____				
_____				
_____				
_____				

FLEXIBILITY, RELAXATION, MEDITATION

	Duration	Cal. Burned
_____		
_____		

DAILY CALORIES BURNED: _____

CALORIE CALCULATOR

	−		=		−		=	
TOTAL CALORIE INTAKE		TOTAL CALORIES BURNED		NET CALORIES		BMR (Basal Metabolic Rate)		DAILY NET CALORIE GAIN OR LOSS

Energy Level: 1 2 3 4 5 6

Muscle Group Worked: ☐ arms ☐ chest ☐ back ☐ core ☐ thighs ☐ calves

Diet & Workout Notes:

_____

_____

DIET JOURNAL

Day 9

DATE: _____   WEIGHT: _____

🍎 BREAKFAST	Qty.	Calories	Fat	Carbs	Other
_____	___				
_____	___				
_____	___				
_____	___				

➕ SNACK	Qty.	Calories	Fat	Carbs	Other
_____	___				

🍔 LUNCH	Qty.	Calories	Fat	Carbs	Other
_____	___				
_____	___				
_____	___				
_____	___				

🍓 SNACK	Qty.	Calories	Fat	Carbs	Other
_____	___				

🥄 DINNER	Qty.	Calories	Fat	Carbs	Other
_____	___				
_____	___				
_____	___				
_____	___				

DAILY INTAKE TOTALS:

✓ **Water Intake**
# of 8 oz. glasses

☐ ☐ ☐
☐ ☐ ☐
☐ ☐ ☐

Daily # of Servings

fruits	meats & beans
veggies	milk & dairy
grains	oils & sweets

Vitamins & Supplements:

_____
_____
_____

FITNESS JOURNAL

DAILY GOAL: _____ GOAL MET: ☐

🏃 CARDIOVASCULAR EXERCISE

	Duration	Distance	Pace	Cal. Burned
_____				
_____				
_____				

🏋 STRENGTH TRAINING

	Weight	Reps.	Sets	Cal. Burned
_____				
_____				
_____				
_____				
_____				
_____				

方 FLEXIBILITY, RELAXATION, MEDITATION

	Duration	Cal. Burned
_____		
_____		

DAILY CALORIES BURNED:

CALORIE CALCULATOR

	−		=		−		=	
TOTAL CALORIE INTAKE		TOTAL CALORIES BURNED		NET CALORIES		BMR (Basal Metabolic Rate)		DAILY NET CALORIE GAIN OR LOSS

Energy Level:
👎 1 2 3 4 5 6 👍

Muscle Group Worked:
☐ arms ☐ chest ☐ back ☐ core ☐ thighs ☐ calves

Diet & Workout Notes:

_____

_____

Day 10 DATE: _____ WEIGHT: _____

BREAKFAST	Qty.	Calories	Fat	Carbs	Other

SNACK	Qty.	Calories	Fat	Carbs	Other

LUNCH	Qty.	Calories	Fat	Carbs	Other

SNACK	Qty.	Calories	Fat	Carbs	Other

DINNER	Qty.	Calories	Fat	Carbs	Other

DAILY INTAKE TOTALS:

✓ **Water Intake**
# of 8 oz. glasses

Daily # of Servings

fruits   meats & beans

veggies   milk & dairy

grains   oils & sweets

Vitamins & Supplements:

FITNESS JOURNAL

DAILY GOAL: _____ GOAL MET: ☐

CARDIOVASCULAR EXERCISE

	Duration	Distance	Pace	Cal. Burned
_____				
_____				
_____				

STRENGTH TRAINING

	Weight	Reps.	Sets	Cal. Burned
_____				
_____				
_____				
_____				
_____				
_____				

FLEXIBILITY, RELAXATION, MEDITATION

	Duration	Cal. Burned
_____		
_____		

DAILY CALORIES BURNED: _____

CALORIE CALCULATOR

	−		=		−		=	
TOTAL CALORIE INTAKE		TOTAL CALORIES BURNED		NET CALORIES		BMR (Basal Metabolic Rate)		DAILY NET CALORIE GAIN OR LOSS

Energy Level:
1 2 3 4 5 6

Muscle Group Worked:
☐ arms ☐ chest ☐ back ☐ core ☐ thighs ☐ calves

Diet & Workout Notes:

_____

_____

Day 11   DATE: _____   WEIGHT: _____

BREAKFAST	Qty.	Calories	Fat	Carbs	Other

SNACK	Qty.	Calories	Fat	Carbs	Other

LUNCH	Qty.	Calories	Fat	Carbs	Other

SNACK	Qty.	Calories	Fat	Carbs	Other

DINNER	Qty.	Calories	Fat	Carbs	Other

DAILY INTAKE TOTALS:

✓ **Water Intake**
# of 8 oz. glasses

☐ ☐ ☐
☐ ☐ ☐

Daily # of Servings

fruits   meats & beans

veggies   milk & dairy

grains   oils & sweets

Vitamins & Supplements:

_____
_____
_____

FITNESS JOURNAL

DAILY GOAL:_____ GOAL MET: ☐

🏃 CARDIOVASCULAR EXERCISE	Duration	Distance	Pace	Cal. Burned

🏋 STRENGTH TRAINING	Weight	Reps.	Sets	Cal. Burned

🧘 FLEXIBILITY, RELAXATION, MEDITATION	Duration	Cal. Burned

DAILY CALORIES BURNED.

CALORIE CALCULATOR

TOTAL CALORIE INTAKE	−	TOTAL CALORIES BURNED	=	NET CALORIES	−	BMR (Basal Metabolic Rate)	=	DAILY NET CALORIE GAIN OR LOSS

Energy Level:
👎 1 2 3 4 5 6 👍

Muscle Group Worked:
☐ arms ☐ chest ☐ back ☐ core ☐ thighs ☐ calves

Diet & Workout Notes:

_____

_____

Day 12

DATE: _____   WEIGHT: _____

BREAKFAST	Qty.	Calories	Fat	Carbs	Other

SNACK	Qty.	Calories	Fat	Carbs	Other

LUNCH	Qty.	Calories	Fat	Carbs	Other

SNACK	Qty.	Calories	Fat	Carbs	Other

DINNER	Qty.	Calories	Fat	Carbs	Other

DAILY INTAKE TOTALS:

✓ **Water Intake**
# of 8 oz. glasses

☐ ☐ ☐
☐ ☐ ☐
☐ ☐ ☐

Daily # of Servings

	fruits		meats & beans
	veggies		milk & dairy
	grains		oils & sweets

Vitamins & Supplements:

_____
_____
_____

FITNESS JOURNAL

DAILY GOAL:_____ GOAL MET: ☐

CARDIOVASCULAR EXERCISE	Duration	Distance	Pace	Cal. Burned

STRENGTH TRAINING	Weight	Reps.	Sets	Cal. Burned

FLEXIBILITY, RELAXATION, MEDITATION	Duration	Cal. Burned

DAILY CALORIES BURNED:

CALORIE CALCULATOR

	−		=		−		=
TOTAL CALORIE INTAKE		TOTAL CALORIES BURNED		NET CALORIES		BMR (Basal Metabolic Rate)	DAILY NET CALORIE GAIN OR LOSS

Energy Level:
👎 1 2 3 4 5 6 👍

Muscle Group Worked:
☐ arms ☐ chest ☐ back ☐ core ☐ thighs ☐ calves

Diet & Workout Notes:

_____

_____

Day 13

DATE:_____   WEIGHT:_____

BREAKFAST	Qty.	Calories	Fat	Carbs	Other

SNACK	Qty.	Calories	Fat	Carbs	Other

LUNCH	Qty.	Calories	Fat	Carbs	Other

SNACK	Qty.	Calories	Fat	Carbs	Other

DINNER	Qty.	Calories	Fat	Carbs	Other

DAILY INTAKE TOTALS:

✓ **Water Intake**
# of 8 oz. glasses

Daily # of Servings

	fruits		meats & beans
	veggies		milk & dairy
	grains		oils & sweets

Vitamins & Supplements:

_____

_____

_____

FITNESS JOURNAL

DAILY GOAL:_____ GOAL MET: ☐

🏃 CARDIOVASCULAR EXERCISE

	Duration	Distance	Pace	Cal. Burned

🏋 STRENGTH TRAINING

	Weight	Reps.	Sets	Cal. Burned

🧘 FLEXIBILITY, RELAXATION, MEDITATION

	Duration	Cal. Burned

DAILY CALORIES BURNED:

CALORIE CALCULATOR

TOTAL CALORIE INTAKE	−	TOTAL CALORIES BURNED	=	NET CALORIES	−	BMR (Basal Metabolic Rate)	=	DAILY NET CALORIE GAIN OR LOSS

Energy Level: 👎 1 2 3 4 5 6 👍

Muscle Group Worked: ☐ arms ☐ chest ☐ back ☐ core ☐ thighs ☐ calves

Diet & Workout Notes:

_____

_____

Day 14   DATE: _____   WEIGHT: _____

BREAKFAST	Qty.	Calories	Fat	Carbs	Other

SNACK	Qty.	Calories	Fat	Carbs	Other

LUNCH	Qty.	Calories	Fat	Carbs	Other

SNACK	Qty.	Calories	Fat	Carbs	Other

DINNER	Qty.	Calories	Fat	Carbs	Other

DAILY INTAKE TOTALS:

✓ **Water Intake**
# of 8 oz. glasses

◯ ◯ ◯
◯ ◯ ◯

Daily # of Servings

fruits   meats & beans

veggies   milk & dairy

grains   oils & sweets

Vitamins & Supplements:
_____
_____
_____

FITNESS JOURNAL

DAILY GOAL: _____ — GOAL MET: ☐

🏃 CARDIOVASCULAR EXERCISE

	Duration	Distance	Pace	Cal. Burned

🏋 STRENGTH TRAINING

	Weight	Reps.	Sets	Cal. Burned

🤸 FLEXIBILITY, RELAXATION, MEDITATION

	Duration	Cal. Burned

DAILY CALORIES BURNED: _____

CALORIE CALCULATOR

TOTAL CALORIE INTAKE	−	TOTAL CALORIES BURNED	=	NET CALORIES	−	BMR (Basal Metabolic Rate)	=	DAILY NET CALORIE GAIN OR LOSS

Energy Level: 👎 1 2 3 4 5 6 👍

Muscle Group Worked: ☐ arms ☐ chest ☐ back ☐ core ☐ thighs ☐ calves

Diet & Workout Notes:

_____

_____

Tell Us Your Weight-Loss Success Story!

We love hearing when our readers successfully lose weight or clothing sizes in just two weeks!

Please tell us your story, your initial weight and measurements, your expectations for this diet and fitness program, etc. Tell us what you liked or didn't like about this book, and what you found useful or wished we had included. Now, tell us how you feel with your new slimmer and healthier body. Share your best advice for others who are struggling with their weight.

Please include the following information:

- Your name:
- Phone number:
- E-mail:
- Your story!
- Before and After photos, if possible

Please email this information to info@WSPublishingGroup.com or send a letter to WS Publishing Group, 15373 Innovation Drive, Suite 360; San Diego, CA 92128.